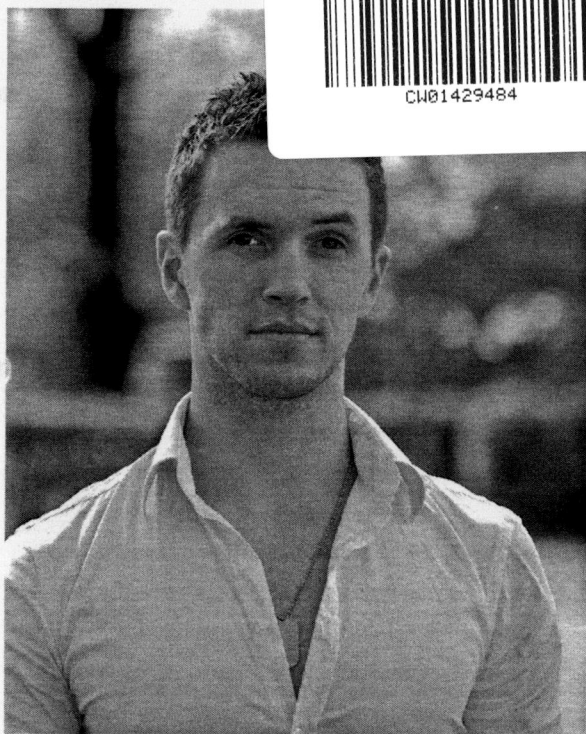

Scott has been involved in the fitness industry for just over 15 years and specialises in Pilates. He is based in London and teaches in a variety of health clubs and corporate settings. He is currently working on his third book, *Pilates For Eternal Youth.*

Don't Push Me

SCOTT GRAHAM

Don't Push Me

'Surviving the fitness industry!
When you love doing what you hate being!'

Vanguard Press

VANGUARD PAPERBACK

© Copyright 2015
Scott Graham

The right of Scott Graham to be identified as author of
this work has been asserted by him in accordance with the
Copyright, Designs and Patents Act 1988.

ISBN 978 178465 068 1

Vanguard Press is an imprint of
Pegasus Elliot MacKenzie Publishers Ltd.
www.pegasuspublishers.com

First Published in 2015

Vanguard Press
Sheraton House Castle Park
Cambridge England

Printed & Bound in Great Britain

Acknowledgements

Spending years in an industry I once despised, I'm grateful to have met the volume of characters who have enlightened and developed me into the fitness professional I am today! As with any industry where people are involved, there are many walks of life. With fitness, I've come across the passionate, the driven, the egotistical, the clueless, the comedians to the absolute sons of bitches – all of whom have inspired me to write this book about the highs and lows of the fitness industry. Special thanks to Stacey Lagonell, Margo Bovell, Michele Hart, Bonnie Toward, Kate Gaunt, Diego Avila, David Anderson, Claire Peacock, Nichola Broadwell and that bitch in Walworth Road. The people and their actions are what make fitness truly an experience worth being involved in.

Contents

FOREWORD

Growing up has its challenges. When a decision has to be made upon what direction to take for a career, there are those who annoyingly know exactly what they want to do, and then there are those who fly head first through the doors of their very first job not knowing what they're about to experience! Mention the word 'fitness' and you just have to look around to see that the majority of people fear they'll be roped into some intensive six-week boot camp course!

Follow the true story of a passionate fitness hater who entered the fitness industry as a result of persistent backache, grew to have a love-hate relationship with the politics of gym life and now reveals to the outsider what goes on behind the mask of an instructor and personal trainer with an inside look at the fitness industry. Whether you're planning to join the industry as a personal trainer or group fitness professional, you're a regular gym goer or simply have a gym phobia then read on to learn what the fitness industry truly has to offer!

CHAPTER ONE

JUST BREATHE!

So the person next to me is groaning with pleasure or is it sighing with relief. An 'in the moment experience' or perhaps a cry for attention! Surely she's going to come round and tell this annoying bitch to shut the fuck up! I mean, the girl has her ass in the air like some satellite dish searching for reception, knees clamped to her ears in some new 'Kama Sutra' position with eyes bulging from sockets. It can't be good for you! At what point in your life do you want to be able to do that? OK, there could be many arguments for it, especially the ones where it's supposedly good for you.

So I'm embracing my new surroundings, the heat, the positions and the smells. My first yogic experience accompanied with surrounding vocalised harmonies. The instructor floated around the room as if high on ecstasy and spoke in a language that was fit for a gardener – 'plant your foot into the floor, blossom at the top and hold your trunk strong in tree pose'. What the hell was she talking about? What had she been smoking? All that was missing was the gardening gloves. I wonder if 'falling tree' or 'tree with branches in distress' are poses. Balancing wasn't easy, but I guess that was the challenge.

I was up close and personal with complete strangers. I couldn't help but notice my neighbours: the attention seekers formally known as the drama queens, the stressed, the disgruntled, the creatures of habit, the desperate housewife, the fashionista, the aspiring yoga teacher wannabe, the introvert, the husband and wife and I. What am I doing with my life? Will I ever decide on a job, a career? When will she hurry the fuck up and tell us to come out of 'tree pose'? My ankles were swelling to trunk like proportions as we held for what seemed like an eternity and my foot felt as if surrounded in weeds. Well, I hope it was weeds otherwise my mat hadn't been cleaned since the last time. If I wanted my feet flossed, I would've gone to the podiatrist! Throughout the class, I did everything the instructor asked of me. I inhaled when told to do so. I exhaled to relax deeper into the pose. At the end of the session, I then started to breathe normally after what seemed like an hour of hyperventilating! Gasping through my mouth and blowing out my ass at the same time!

I guess there's a reason why it's called mind and body! The positions were excruciatingly barbaric for my body. Every move contorted me in ways that brought fear to my mind. Once in these positions, would I ever get out of them? Would I end up with my leg mangled around my waist until I could afford reconstructive surgery to dislodge my dislocated joints? The instructor, when demonstrating the moves, did so with grace and elegance. Her face was noticeably calm. When I glanced in the mirror at myself, I looked as if I was chewing a wasp.

The formula of people and positions brought an array of smells to my sensitive nose. Garlic bread from the night before intensified with each breath out from the perpetrators mouth. Morning breath from a non-brushed mouth placed extra havoc to my wasp-ravaged facial expression. If the smell wasn't coming from one end, it was certainly seeping through from the other. If it wasn't the noise that alarmed the ears of the unconscious, it was the odour, which could certainly awaken even the dead. I'd recommend perhaps a change of diet especially cutting out baked beans before a stint in yoga. The atmosphere smelt like some new-style recipe I didn't want to sample. As for sweat, well, let's just say it gives you away every time. Whether it be the alcohol or curry from the night before or something more natural like the smell of the sweat in the first place, it made me question why I didn't try the DVD option from the comforts of home in the first instance! Lying face down on the mat made me think of cheese sandwiches and onion bagels, or at least that's what my nose sensed as I planted my face into the mat whilst trying to lift my legs off the floor. At key points in the class, I found myself plotting my escape plan. With each upside-down pose, I thought while nobody's looking I could tiptoe through the sweaty people to return my mat. I could reach my final destination, a place similar to heaven, a place where people could breathe in fresh air and eat doughnuts! Scared to commit a crime against the laws of yoga, I was frozen in place or in some cases cemented like some paving slab. I was unable to move with no idea how to get out from some of the positions. The one-hour session came to an end, and I was impressed with myself for achieving, staying and persevering throughout the trauma of movement and smell. I have to confess I did feel better afterwards. I felt loose in places I never knew I could be with a face like a stoned cat!

My constant backache had forced me to try the things I thought I'd never do. Yoga! YOGA! I couldn't even touch my toes but who cares, that's why we have knees, right? At that point in time, my concept of exercise was walking from bedroom to kitchen and back to bedroom again. I needed food to survive and was told that rest was good for me! OK, I needed to change my thought process on exercise. After all, spending my entire life at secondary school avoiding physical education had eventually taken its toll. Saying that, at school, if you weren't into football or rugby, you were pretty much screwed. Besides, being lined up, as if for an execution, to be selected by the top sportsmen of the year, and then to be finally shot third from last wasn't my idea of a confidence booster. So I guess I could pinpoint my backache from here on; permanent and progressive – or at least that's what the mirror told me. Strangely my back seemed phobic at the thought of taking part in physical education at school. Was it the aggression and lack of enthusiasm in doing rugby or was it the people in my class that had made my mind up? The competitive streak of some guys can be their way of saying that they have not been blessed in the downstairs department; therefore they need to prove their worth through their physical demeanour! Whatever the reason, the lack of variety we were given to choose from: football, rugby, rugby or football inspired me as much as a rocket to my ass would have!

School's in the past thankfully, and uni life was exciting and liberating. The people, the lectures, the drink and the freedom! My hormones were raging, and my male urge to become manlier was coursing through me. I wanted a sports car, but my bank account struggled to pay the bus fare. I resorted towards my second ambition – get muscles! Uni had a different atmosphere to it. Whether it was age or uni, I felt more encouraged to actually try the whole exercise thing.

DAY ONE AT THE GYM!

Approaching a gym, never mind joining the gym, was a daunting experience. Paying for something which caused pain was utter madness, but my first attempt to gain muscle by drinking protein powder just didn't work. I was baffled! I read the label and regularly drank these protein shakes as required. Having at least one shake a day, if not twice, should've done the job, but instead of increased muscle size,

I had an increased usage of toilet paper. If it wasn't blocking toilets via my belly, it was my belly itself which felt bloated and my self-esteem deflated, just like my muscles. I felt cheated, the magazines I read made the claims that I could achieve a six-pack in seven days. I now know what they were actually meaning to say was that after you take a picture of yourself, spend the next seven days on Photoshop editing out the flabby parts and doctoring it so that a six-pack will show. I just needed to figure out how to make myself look a little more bronzed, but perhaps that was in the second edition which I probably didn't read properly either. After the protein trials and in-depth magazine analysis, I finally concluded with my deluded mind that actually lifting weights was the answer!

To start my new fitness regime, the fitness consultant, Paul, had managed to coerce me into participating in their fitness test. I thought it was a great place to begin my journey, or so I was brainwashed into thinking. Paul had the classic 'Men's Health' magazine front cover body. His biceps could crack walnuts as he flexed his arms giving me an inferiority complex! His bulging chest, similar to his ego, a little overinflated, looked as if he should be wearing a bra. As he stood next to me, it made me feel like I should start shopping at the toddlers' section for my next T-shirt! The teenager in me, however, arrogantly believed, with youth on my side, the fitness test should be a walk in the park.

The test began, and throughout I whimpered pathetically: a running machine, a squeezy machine, reaching a box, a breath test, body measurements and a few other contraptions. Before the test commenced, body measurements were taken. This had the desired effect of highlighting that my arms were just slightly bigger than that of a pen. I was slim with very little fat, little muscle but a lot of hope! The blood-pressure machine seemed to have a mind of its own as it slowly crushed my arm to death with the intention of draining the blood out through my fingertips. The results were all noted down, and to complete the body measurements, I was then asked to blow into a tube. The peak-flow instrument measured lung capacity, which made me question the relevance of it; after all, I only had to blow out candles once a year.

I began the one-hour test on the treadmill, well, not quite the whole hour but the five-minute test made it feel as if I was trekking halfway over the continent. Checking to see if I had a heart and lungs, I certainly discovered I could sweat as my legs quivered in fear with the stress placed on them. I could picture myself like some Pac-Man game – collecting dots, mouth opened and taking everything in except oxygen. As long as my legs could carry me from the house to the local convenience store and back again, my legs hadn't been challenged in such a way before. After my marathon, it was time to test my strength. A weird contraption with a dial on it was used to gauge if I really was Superman. I was directed to hold it out to the side of my body, parallel to my shoulder, and then as I lowered the machine towards my hip, I had to squeeze two bars together. After what I thought was a valiant effort, I was asked to repeat the exercise! Offended by this request, I wanted to reach for his two bars in the form of the sides of his neck and squeeze hard but instead calmly asked through gritted teeth if it was normal to repeat the test. With some of the tests, it was necessary to perform them three times to get an average score, so thankfully it quashed my insecurity of being able to snap a pencil in two. Like analysing a flight attendant, I watched the instructor's face during my fitness assessment to see if there were any changes in his facial expression. His looks of concern and anxiety would panic me. Was I bad? Was I shit? The psychologist in me tried to analyse his thought patterns. I couldn't tell with his 'Mona Lisa' expression. Was he happy? Was he shocked?

The next test consisted of a box with numbers on it, otherwise known as the stretch test. I was instructed to sit on the floor, legs extended, and feet against the box with my back upright. The instructor told me to tip forwards and reach as far as I could. Little did he realise, but I was already trying to reach for the box before he even told me to start. My fingers were steadily growing from my hands as I magically wiggled them closer to the box to at least get some form of measurement. Where are Freddy Krueger's knife gloves when you need them? The back of my legs felt strangled with loss of sensation to my feet. My hamstrings were about to pop. My neck grew like 'E.T.' as I thrusted my head forward making my eyes bulge from their sockets and giving me the impression I was closer to the box.

Instructed to breathe out as I reached forwards, I groaned as if I'd been constipated for a week. After the third attempt, I felt my last vein in my forehead explode, and the back of my legs seemed to have smoke slowly billowing from them like burning frayed wires. Who would have thought stretching to be a workout in itself? Call the fire brigade!

With the test complete, I was impressed to receive a booklet for my efforts. As I eagerly glanced through each page, I was perplexed with the red-like bar charts. The consultant systematically flicked through the pages describing to me in what I now see as a politically correct way of describing 'your fitness is shit'! The red squares in the bar charts highlighted 'danger, you're going to die'! Well, not quite, but the thought of being told I was poor at everything made me ponder over what the cancellation policy for the gym would be. The gym was great at promoting its services, but right at that moment I felt a counselling service would've benefited my self-acceptance of how feeble I was.

The next day, like a cheese grater to the balls, I grudgingly went to the gym to enrol on yet another gym product, as advised by Paul (aka Satan). This time, Boot Camp for six weeks! It was a small group of about twelve and a mixture of girls and guys. We started with the warm-up, which I swear felt like the workout. It was vigorous and intense and to my relief and dedicated skills towards clock watching no more than an hour. We moved around various stations to punish the body in different ways. I looked around the room to see how the rest of the group was coping. Everyone seemed focused and resilient. The instructor told us to work to our own level, but, being male, you can't help but compete with the other guys. After the session, I hit the shower, not physically, but literally speaking! Although my body wanted to hit the floor, I felt that I had abused it enough, so any more physical trauma to it was a definite no-no. The shower-gel dispensers were too high for me to reach, even though before the session they were in the perfect place. Bending my arm reminded my brain of what happened the last time I did that, and so my brain communicated to my arm to not go there again! Thank God for elbows! As for trying to wash my hair, well, the intention was there, but I quickly decided to save that for perhaps later in the week!

The following morning, I had the day off from uni. One of those glorious study days, which are really designed for detoxing from the night before, however, not so much a glory on this day. My body lay in bed paralysed with aches that I'd never experienced before. Well, at least it detracted from the usual backache. Would I ever move again? I needed a defibrillator to restart my heart and to get my body to move. Eventually rolling out of bed about midday, I trudged through to have breakfast. Eating breakfast would've been easier if it had been made for me. Eating breakfast would've been easier if I didn't have to use my arms to lift the spoon and perhaps use a straw instead to suck the porridge from the bowl. After strategically eating breakfast, I felt in order to be more humanlike I ought to get changed. Getting changed was a workout in itself. T-shirt and jeans, hmmm, perhaps not the T-shirt. Lifting my arms away from the sides of my body required muscles that at this moment in time were on strike. A clothing strategy was required, and a shirt was the only viable option to minimise discomfort, although wearing a cloak from last Halloween would've reduced my arm and body movement, and, of course, would've been the best option if it wasn't summer.

Four days later, like a person due for tooth extraction, I returned to Boot Camp having missed one session. I was still tender and forced to scuff my feet across the ground as lifting my heels off the floor caused too much discomfort to my lower legs, thighs and facial muscles. I convinced Paul, the instructor, that I was still too physically challenged to make any kind of movement apart from blinking after the first session, and he prescribed – yoga! It's true what Elton John sings; there definitely is a circle of life. The weeks passed, and coupled with the boot camp sessions, I tried yoga for a second time. It would help me limber up the tightness I'd created through circuit training and help me achieve an upright posture from the 'L' position I'd been exhibiting lately from all the dead lifting. I felt the 'burn' with everyone's 'no pain, no gain' approach, but at some point surely the 'burn' dissipates to something a little cooler, more comfortable and eventually the ability to walk normally without turning heads. Will sitting on the toilet ever become easier without the use of a wall to climb down, sigh?

YOGA ROUND TWO!

I was running late for round two of yoga. Everyone was in class and they'd already started. I felt the pressure already, should I enter the room? Seriously, never mess with the creatures of habit. These people, with their rituals and routines, arrive super early for class, mat clamped under their arms as if to go to war, march in to claim their 'spot' in the studio of which heaven forbid you steal their space. For the yogis who are supposed to be calm, relaxed and chilled, they must be the most highly-strung people I've come across – and breathe. I hesitated outside the studio doors for a short time wondering, fearing and analysing! Would I become one of these creatures, or was it a dormant fear of being surrounded with them yet again? I took a deep breath in, and as I breathed out, opened the door.

During yoga, we were in a seated position, legs out in front, reaching for our toes. At this moment in time, I had a flashback to the killer stretch test. My spine wouldn't bend. I felt and looked like I had a non-bendy rod down my back making me look constipated as I tipped forwards. I started reminiscing back to the fitness test. There must be some form of spinal fusion running the length of my spine, either that or I was as flexible as concrete. I'm not that tall, but when doing some of these stretches, I wished for shorter legs or arms at least twice as long. Even the pregnant woman next to me was touching her toes. How on earth is that possible? To make matters worse, next to super gran was bendy grandad with the tightest pants I've witnessed since watching the Olympic sprinters run. How can he breathe in those spandex hot pants, eurgh! I tried to duck my head down to at least look like I was bending forward, you know, blend into the class. I heard the teacher instruct, using her gardening language, for us all to not force the stretch, although her tone sounded like it was directed to me. Just looking at my toes with the contemplation of 'one day my finger nail will touch my toe if I grow them long enough' was a push too far. I spied from the corner of my eye that annoying yoga bitch that was in the yoga class the first time I was there. She was right at the front. She puts the itch in bitch. A scratch in the back you just can't reach. It just lingers. A wannabe! Is she training to be a yoga teacher as she certainly looked like she was taking the class? Maybe she's a dancer or an attention-starved housewife. Oh well, I couldn't help but smirk at grumpy grandma for her disapproving glares at the two giggling high school girls at the back. Why is it some yogis just can't be content within themselves and ignore what's happening around them, and as for others, they look like they need a nice fattening cheeseburger every once in a while? Some look so fragile they're going to break! Focus, must focus!

Executing the moves throughout the class was an uphill struggle although I managed to perform them silently, unlike others. Expressive groans, like giving birth or as if vinegar had been rubbed into a gaping wound in the privates, were heard throughout the studio. Is it really necessary? Is it the attention seekers calling for the spotlight to shine on them? Is it the praise seekers looking for affirmation from the instructor that they are doing the moves wonderfully well? Some people's idea of breathing can be vocally dramatised like some perverted old man preying over some younger model but without the drool. Well, in some cases there can be involuntary drool left lying on the floor, which, without fail, my foot manages to find with ease! Breathing out can be heavy, deep, prolonged and generally over-exaggerated as if someone has consumed too many chillies, HAAAAAAAAAAA!

At the end of the class, there was ten minutes of relaxation. Ten minutes of lying on the mat, relaxing in 'corpse pose'. My favourite pose to do. Lie there motionless and I'm sure the real reason why most people come to class is for the simple excuse that they can say to others that they've been to yoga. Some people in class looked dead, I felt dead, and now we had the opportunity to play dead! The instructor told me I was particularly good at this pose. Sarcastic bitch! The lights were dimmed, and the soft music echoed out from the stereo. The teacher's soft tones, similar to that of a sex-telephone operator, hypnotised the guy next to me who purred with a subtle snore of contentment. Relaxation is such a difficult thing to do. My mind's actively thinking about where I should go at the weekend, the lecture I did in the morning and the assignment that I needed to pull together for a week's time. What do I want to do for a career? Will I ever be rich and why was this guy's snoring sounding rather like a song I heard on the radio the morning before? Concentrate! I must learn to concentrate. Oh, and relax! Throughout the session my back was starting to feel less like a ninety-year-old man and more like the teenager I was. Coupled with the fact of feeling limber and more energised, all that I knew at this point in time was a slight addiction to this fitness malarkey and that I could start to see a small lump popping through in the form of a muscle, or was it wishful thinking (or even a tumour)?

AFTER UNI...

Time eroded quickly, and before I knew it I'd finished uni and had achieved my combined studies Master's degree in Advanced Psychology, Strategic Marketing and International Relations. How useful would I be to the world now? To follow on from my uni qualification, I decided to study a fitness instructor course, not really knowing which direction to take. A feeling of 'shit, I need to be an adult now and find a job!' Like many graduates, the next step in life was to do something completely different to what had been studied over the years. Master's then fitness! Do the two go together? The two are linked: it's studying, requires effort and commitment and yes, I guess I was still clueless with what I wanted to do with my life. Everyone at school had everything mapped out. They will be this, do that and have the family by then. How organised, how focused, how sad! Was I just rebelling against the norm, or did I just need a little more time to think about things? Maybe a few more relaxation sessions at the end of yoga would get things into perspective. I really did despise secondary school and many of the people that came with it. Teenagers are funny creatures; hormones raging with this common ideology of falling into a great job after school because they've studied hard and achieved a grade one or a pass with merit. I hate the small-town mentality and even their idea of exercise is different to mine. If they offered weight training at PE instead of sports, perhaps, I would have taken part in something that I actually didn't completely suck at. Maybe I'd be the lead guy up at the front of the class choosing who I felt was good enough to be in my team, relishing the part where I select those who need to be shot because of their worthlessness. Harsh I know, but I'm just embracing the evil thought as I'm sure they did. After leaving school, my training and studying came together for the fact I actually started to learn something and that the gym was not as intimidating as I first envisaged. Who would have thought that I'd embrace the fitness culture! It's funny, but I felt I'd learnt more after leaving school than I did in all of my younger years!

I studied the fitness instructor course through open learning so that I could start making money for the sports car that I so desired. I find learning beyond a classroom atmosphere sometimes really can be the best way to learn. It avoids being surrounded by idiots who ask questions that defy logic! I wanted to learn about fitness for my personal gain. I had a desire to improve my body with no intention of actually becoming an instructor! During the course, I was working part-time in a supermarket as a shelf replenishment officer or SRO for short. The job entailed stock control, rotation, replenishment, advertising of promotions and many other demandingly fancy titles. I guess the 'real' title that most people assign to the job is shelf stacker! I just couldn't come to call it that, and in order to keep my social status looking cool, I was an SRO who would stack shelves in a coordinated, strategic manner requiring years of experience and training that only a few elite people could do! Also for the fact that I thought maybe one day I'd lose my interest in fitness, not find a job with my degree and need to continue this job role on a full-time basis until I decided what direction to take. I contemplated a role as a section manager, looking after a department within the supermarket but soon realised that I was clutching at ideas for potential jobs to gain some direction in life! There are only so many cans of beans you can stack on a shelf before knowing the nutritional content per bean and in the process talking in some form of bean language. Small-town, supermarket mentality was tiring but amusing all the same. Vera, Stefan and Melissa, my work colleagues, otherwise known as the gossipmongers, would start or stop discussing me as soon as I either left or entered the room. I guess I felt privileged and honoured that their time could be taken up with issues involving me, as I'm sure they did with many others. The gossip, a fulfilment in their lives and I thank them for that, fuelled me to strive for greater ambition within myself. Maybe SRO wasn't the way forward! I didn't want to be in a job where I found myself complaining about it like the others and not change my circumstances. Seeing the evolution of bean-can labelling changing as the years pass by! Doomed to complain and moan about the same job in years to come. ARGH! Time will tell, actions speak louder!

I finished the instructor course in six months having collected one huge son-of-a-bitch folder full of papers, notes and coffee stains. Having finished the course with a three-day exam, my mind was bursting full of knowledge on how to keep fit, and I was eager and ready to share this abundance of information with the world. I felt inspired, motivated and thirsty for more input – need more input, like Short Circuit (the film). I started researching into the possibility of entering the fitness industry as an instructor and this soon paved the way to the start of my journey.

CHAPTER TWO

LET'S INSTRUCT!

The day finally arrived when I emigrated from the small town of Forfar in Scotland to the city of Dundee. So maybe the words not quite emigrate, as Forfar to Dundee is only a twenty-minute drive from each other, however, to me the move was one big step for mankind from a town I felt was trapped in a time warp to a city that offered hope and progression. I moved into my first, ridiculously cheap bought pad, a one-bedroomed 'homely' flat (homely as in small but neat). The smaller the place the less cleaning needed, and besides, a clean house is a sign of a wasted life. Oh, the parties I had in that place must've pissed the neighbours off, but hey, I hope they understood life is for living! I have to admit though the next morning when I had to cautiously carry a bin bag full of clattering bottles down one flight of stairs in fear of arousing the neighbours, made me feel like I had a drink problem. Oh, the youth of today! The move to Dundee was solely for the purpose of being closer to my new place of work and to get away from the dregs.

The beginning of my first full time job as a fitness instructor at Relish Fitness was amazing. I met the manager and the small team of fellow instructors. Bonnie, I could tell just connected with me. Her focus, drive and direction inspired me. In fact they were all motivational and driven individuals. Just what I needed surrounding me after my part-time job at the local supermarket. Optimistic souls in comparison from the soulless individuals I had the 'fortune' to work with!

The gym was small with a few treadmills, bikes and some prehistoric 'Fred Flintstone' weight machines that creaked with every movement, or maybe the noise was stemming from the people who seemed as happy as a pig, not in shit, but frozen in time and place. Everything was new and exciting, but it didn't take long before it felt more like visiting an old-folks home with resentment and the belief that you'd be faced with the same routine, same conversations and surrounding smells!

There came a time, a few months working for Relish Fitness, that I started to complain about the monotony of the role. Life as a fitness instructor wasn't as glam as I had imagined, in fact it was tedious. I was cleaning frigging machines after sweaty runners had projected their drool everywhere. Vile! I was trying to create a persona of professionalism to reflect my newfound knowledge of fitness. Cleaning wasn't something I had a phobia for, but I felt the cleaning side of it should've been left to the experts in cleaning. Call me a snob, but when I was on the other side as 'the member' I wanted the person who was coaching, inspiring and motivating me to do so through my perception of what an instructor was supposed to do, and that was to instruct, not put the marigolds on and start scrubbing! Half the time, I felt the pressure imposed on cleaning would soon result in me sticking a broom up my ass whilst carrying out an induction! Kill two birds with one stone or mop two bikes with one swoop! I didn't want to wake up forcing a passion on myself and the thought process of 'mmm, I can't wait to get in there and clean those fucking machines raw. Who's been a dirty machine then!' Out with the vacuum, on with the marigolds. I'd not long finished a degree and I was cleaning machines, why bother with the degree! It was my first job so I had to come to terms by giving myself a pep talk about the deluded expectations I had from doing a degree. What was I expecting? Leaving uni to walk into an executive fitness instructor role, leather chair with big fat-ass cigar in mouth. OK, it's fitness, maybe not the cigar, a fruit juice perhaps. Earning from a full-time job felt great. I was a grown-up. The money, however, never seemed to fill my bank account the way I wanted it to. What can I expect from a job though! After all, doesn't JOB stand for 'Just Over Broke'? I was certainly living my life through JOB!

The manager, Gillian, seemed intimidated by me for wanting to make a change, make a difference within the working role. I listed, through my enthusiasm, the possibilities to her, what we could introduce to the member, how we could generate revenue and make the job one full of passion. She responded with half-hearted replies and excuses of not having the budget or the finances. 'Manage for crying out loud!' as I grabbed her and shook her, slapping her either side of the face – 'MANAGE!' Dreaming was as far as I would get with her. Dreaming that one day we would get progression within the work place, or perhaps that I would actually grab her and slap her with passion for a place I saw potential in. Give me strength, surely if you're time has expired, and you're bored of the job, move on and don't drag us all into the depths of despair.

Grant, alias protein boy, was part of the fitness team. He was a big friendly giant whose concept of putting on muscle size was devouring as much protein as was humanly possible. He had the bulk but was more muscle than brain, or should I say more protein than muscle. He had obviously taken steroids in the past but openly admitted it as if it were some kind of accolade to be proud of. I was convinced that behind closed doors he probably kissed his arms regularly; in some momentous glory to self-congratulate his achievement. Grant loved being 'the Hulk'. What the hell, I'm sure I can recall once or twice when he kissed 'his guns' on the gym floor, in front of members. Cringe! What do some of these members think about some of these morons who are acting as professionals? All beef, no brains!

It was evident to those in the know when Grant was on his course of 'roids.' His water-retentive muscles, bad skin and shiny forehead, which shone in your face like car headlights to a rabbit, were key signs to stay away, roid rage on tour. The spots on his back were pulsing full of puss, enough to fill a shot glass. Like other steroid users, it was advised that if they're on the 'gear', stay clear. These highly fuelled and testosterone overloaded guys would lose their temper at the slightest of things. 'Hi, how you doing?' Swoop! Wow all I said was 'hi!' Perhaps it's not how it's said, maybe it's the way it's been said, that grates on these over-sensitive beasts.

I was on shifts, which meant I didn't get the opportunity to get to know the other instructors. Mornings were killers especially during winter and particularly when the gym opened at six thirty in the morning. I'm not a morning person and to be there to greet people with enthusiasm and motivation was a challenge in itself. I thought maybe I should record a really cheery upbeat message, 'hey there, morning, how you doing?' so I could press play each time someone walked through the doors. It would save on my energy for later in the day and making the effort with people who didn't give me the time of day. What really is highly frustrating is when greeting someone and they blatantly ignore you as if you're some piece of shit that happens to be in their way. Hmm, the temptation to actually pull the plug on them when they were running full steam ahead was sometimes a temptation too hard to resist. 'Fly you fucker, FLY! Oh I'm sorry, I didn't mean to switch off your treadmill whilst you were running. It was supposed to be my vacuum!' Even more amusing would be 'accidentally' switching off the treadmill whilst they were running for an hour avidly watching the calorie counter ticking away. 'Oops, sorry again. Really I am!' I don't understand how people want to exercise so early in the morning when they have the enthusiastic look of a hamster to a wheel! I guess the early morning can explain the miserable faces and socially-reclusive lifestyles of some of these hard done by people. Work commitments, I guess, force these early risers to get up so early, or perhaps some fitness addiction or some sordid romantic fling between two married people who can only rendezvous first thing in the empty sauna.

Eating breakfast so early in the morning is a workout for me in itself; trying to keep it down for a starter, especially if I cook scrambled eggs. Even worse if I sleep in and then am forced to shovel it down my throat without chewing in order to fuel me for the day ahead. Maybe it's me with my issue of getting up at ridiculous o'clock that makes me so grumpy. What's even more traumatic is a freezing cold morning. I don't do Eskimos and ice at the best of times.

I lasted about one year at Relish Fitness before I clawed my hair out from early mornings, cleaning and writing the same old boring programmes for people. Weight loss with extra focus on legs and ass was the goal for every woman who came to the gym. Even the skinny girls wanted their legs and ass worked on. I came across some wide-hipped women and would recommend for them to broaden their shoulders to complement their hips especially if they were posturally rounded in their upper torso/shoulder region. I swear some women have ginormous hips to the point that when measuring them, I felt the need to attach a boomerang to the tape measure and swing it around their hips so I could get the whole circumference. It was either that or bear hug them which wasn't the most ethically correct way of doing things. Cheek pressed up against their hip like mother to child while breast feeding – mama! Part of the fitness test involved measurements and at times, I thought does the person I'm measuring really want to be told that there isn't enough tape measure to go around. Even standing on the scales was a nerve-racking experience for both instructor and client. Like watching Titanic with apprehension, how would it all end? Sink or swim? Would there be enough numbers on the scale or was the dial able to turn past 'zero' more than once to get some form of measurement! So I tended to 'selectively' avoid the tape measuring and weighing part to avoid stress on the participant and myself. Unfortunately, some women really do believe that fitness professionals are miracle workers and can help them lose their hips! Two answers for this: surgery or perhaps by finding comfort in taking out a lawsuit against the parents under the pretence of unfair genetics!

From someone who has had first-hand experience in fitness testing, there are for and against arguments to testing. It's great if you're fairly fit and trying to get fitter, but if you're a completely inactive cake lover, it's not going to feel and read great. Imagine turning every page, glaring at the red bar charts advertising a ticking time bomb. Being told you're overweight by enormous proportions, your lung capacity is the size of a hamster and your flexibility could be improved if you purchased one of those grabber sticks to save you bending down to pick up things, or by standing every so often in contrast to a seated position, oh, and avoid eating cake by getting a lock to your fridge or at least get an automatic time lock on your fridge so you don't binge eat after hours!

A STEP UP!

My next fitness role after Relish Fitness was Poser Paradise Gyms. I was hired because of my experience, for the fact I had a K.O.B.O. certificate and simply because they obviously loved me at the interview for my sweet charms, GUSH! It was a step up, more money, more of a challenge and a bigger gym. This gym had an impressively huge studio that catered for around fifty members. Like a kid to a candy shop my eyes lit up seeing the studio as I envisaged myself teaching in front of groups of people. It was a huge contrast to my secondary school life where even the idea of standing in front of the class was a ball-wrenching concept. The gym itself had rows of treadmills, cross-trainers, bikes and rowers. Several TVs hanging from the ceiling in front of all the cardio machines were the prize to entice those eager to train and to bribe those not so keen. Cardio machines have to be the most challenging for not just the body but for the mind. Besides being mind-numbingly boring, it can be rather awkward when running during a busy period and all that's showing on TV is Embarrassing Illnesses. A group of guys getting their testicles checked by doctors and women having utensils inserted into places that make your jaw drop just don't motivate me to run! It's either that or watch the guy run with his hooded top up, the rather large woman drink diet coke while on the bike, or a woman who seems to think the communal spa is for women only, and is wearing nothing apart from a pair of those plastic blue shoes which are for sole use over outdoor trainers in wet areas! My mate, David, who was also a fitness trainer within the club, told the lady in question that it was a spa for both men and women and that the shoes were for using over outdoor trainers. Her reply, she had a verruca and thought it was for that. There are people in the gym that need help and then there are others that need HELP!

There's a completely different vibe in the gym in the morning compared to the evening and this is reflected in the studio too. The morning crowd tend to be the mothers, housewives, unemployed and those retired. From nine thirty to ten thirty the gym and the studio are reasonably busy and afterwards both empty, and the lounge transforms into a coffee morning meeting for the weekly gossip. Exercise is lightly performed with the music softly playing. In the evening, the music is pumping with heavy house beats and techno, busy and buzzing with most machines in use and there's a competitive but friendly feel with fashion, fitness, looks and egos. It's predominantly a younger crowd, and the classes within the studio are electric. Busy classes feed the instructor's motivation, accentuating their ego, which in turn fuels even the less enthusiastic exerciser.

HI, MY NAME IS...

The day nervously came where I had to teach my first ever group fitness class, K.O.B.O (pronounced Ky-bo). This was a mix up of martial arts and aerobics without any set music. Although we received a CD to use for the class during the K.O.B.O. course, the music was undeniably dull. Jungle and bass isn't exactly inspiring music to motivate when working out unless of course you're stoned, wearing earplugs or on strong morphine to numb the pain. So I guess the programme was flawed from the start, but here's little old me standing in front of twenty non-impressionable faces. My manager was also there for a piece of the action and to further intimidate me. I was pouring with sweat before I even started the warm up. Trying to look confident but falling to pieces inside. Having rehearsed a routine leading up to the class, I thought I was prepared. Nothing, however, prepares you for the response, or lack of in this case, when you teach a class. Folded arms, death stares and unmotivated stances waiting in anticipation for what you have to deliver. Come on 'what shit have you got to give us' kind of looks! It looked so easy when I looked through the studio door on several past occasions and saw the instructor effortlessly do their thing. Surely anybody could do this!

The forty-five-minute class lasted an eternity, and when I think about it, I taught a shit class!

Everyone was sweating, so I thought job done, or was it the fact that the heater was accidentally cranked up instead of the fans? I taught the class for a few weeks before I craftily persuaded the management to change the class to something more member pleasing like watching a fitness DVD for an hour, a game of Wii or at least something more comfortable for me to instruct like drinking tea!

Doing the K.O.B.O course whilst working at Relish Fitness was intimidating to say the least. I travelled down to London to do the two-day course. Two lesbianic instructors aggressively taking jabs at everyone on the course instilled a fear of death in me. Please don't cry if she hits you hard, I thought to myself. Thankfully she got so far around the room demonstrating her butch skills to prove a point before she finally ceased her assault and explained the concept of K.O.B.O. I have many lesbian friends but these two were definitely man haters. I'm sure their fists were filled with lead! In the last few years K.O.B.O has been panned for its lack of style and technique in the martial-art field. I have to admit it must be insulting for those martial artists who spend years training and perfecting their art to have followers who teach what they preach over a two-day course. I'd never whacked a punch before the course and have never done so since doing the classes within Poser Paradise Gyms! My 'Mike Tyson' years were short-lived and finally put to bed! K.O.B.O, although another one of those crazy phases in fitness, made me identify that boxing wasn't my thing. I punched like a right bitch and obviously didn't have the inbuilt aggression needed for such a discipline.

JOIN ME FOR A RIDE!

It seemed Poser Paradise Gyms wanted to invest in me as an individual, sending me on my first training course that I'd been on for a long time. 'RPM', part of the Les Mills programmes and the fancily-branded name for cycling on a stationary bike, in the early days had some great music coupled with some great choreography. I really enjoyed it. The workshop lasted two days before attaining certification, and from then we were released into the wild to perform to the multitudes. RPM is a pre-choreographed programme and I started with release twelve. What I hadn't realised was that there were quarterly updates throughout the year to attend in order to renew and refresh the music and the routine (and make Les Mills richer). RPM 12 was the release I started with when I went on the course and had taught one class a week for about four months using the same annoyingly-frustrating, shitty music. At first great, but having learnt the routine over and over, and to then teach it over the period of months you can imagine the songs started to sound as harmonised as a cat on acid. I had resorted to sifting through my own music collection to use in class before the communication finally filtered through that I had to go on a continuing workshop. Release fifteen was a welcome addition to my collection. RPM, unlike K.O.B.O taught me effective ways to teach a class. The essence of pre-cueing, delivery of a safe and enjoyable class along with motivating participants gave me the confidence to get back in the studio and take control. It took a little while to acclimatise to the head mic, which made me feel like some Michael Jackson wannabe, but over time it would become my best friend, saving me from losing my voice from trying to scream at those not paying attention. Like everything, RPM had its shelf life for me, and as the music eventually became more like a country and western / rock concert, I slowly lost interest. It wasn't very inspiring for the crowd I had to teach, and besides paying near enough twenty pounds for a CD whereby only two songs out of the nine were any good was not exactly value for money. I was just waiting for the day when they expected us to race on the bikes with Celine Dion screeching out, 'My heart will go on'! The question was could my legs go on? I stopped attending the RPM quarterly workshops and years later received a letter declaring my decertification, but on the same note if I wanted to continue 'riding a bike' I could redo the course for a reduced rate! Like the vast array of fitness courses on offer, and as I often find out the expensive way, it was a complete money-spinner. Do I really need to re-qualify in how to ride a bike? Am I going to forget what direction the wheels are supposed to turn? Why on earth did they not question why I stopped attending the workshops in the first instance! I'd made up my mind to never get back on the saddle again. It would save me money in the long term and also reduce the increasing friction burns on my inner thighs, forcing me to walk like a cowboy.

The hardest part about teaching a cycle class was when you were not in the mood to motivate but yet were confronted with around twenty faces staring at you expecting a miracle. Unlike mat-based classes, it was not as easy as to have everyone lie face down to hide the misery and despair displayed on some people's faces. The eye-to-eye contact between instructor and member had a look as if to say, 'what the fuck are we doing with our lives'! I recognised the look, as it was the same expression that reflected back to me in the mirror many years prior to teaching! Although an instructor is there for others to follow, there are the few who take it upon themselves to do their own workout and in some cases slap on their iPod and workout to their own music. Am I simply there as a background cabaret act to these people? It's definitely not the easiest job trying to drill motivation through yourself in order to motivate others when you're having an 'off day.' Even worse was during the Christmas period when classes were noticeably quieter. People for some reason like to pack themselves in the back row of the studio, which leaves you looking even more isolated, and in despair on a bike in the front. Move to the front I won't bite, well not yet anyway until you piss me off, and don't you dare look at me in that way! It's not my fault you hate the Christmas hustle and bustle! And smile, composure, let's begin!

GYM, WHO'S JIM?

As I settled into Poser Paradise Gyms' way of life, the fitness instructor role became a little dull and repetitive. Same shit, different location! I was thriving from the classes, but outside the studio there would be a chore of the dreaded cleaning and programme writing, tone up and lose weight blah blah blah. Most of the programmes looked the same – strap yourself to the treadmill and 'run Forest, ruuuuuuuun'. Programmes just don't work in my book. As soon as you shoved somebody on the treadmill (shoved being the operative word), and as soon as your back was turned, they'd be off luxuriating in the spa. Well, I guess you can't make a hamster run the wheel, but don't complain when you haven't lost the weight. What if I pull the plug on the spa – suction so intense that some of these weight-losers fight for their life as they swim to the top? Ta-da congratulations, a new workout created, weight loss achieved and character, strength and development enhanced along the way.

Treadmills, cross trainers and the rest of the cardio machines, normally positioned in long regimented rows, are all tedious contraptions. If you have your own music, it can make the journey a little more durable. Never rely on the music on the treadmills, however, as they always, without fail, never work or it becomes a musical challenge to fill in the blanks during the songs. Tuning into the TV channels can result in listening to Glee while watching some wildlife documentary making you at first feel like the animals are singing whilst you're on some weird acid trip!

There's definitely more of an atmosphere in the studio, everybody working together and of course competing with each other. If not competing with their fitness levels then competing for the latest branded sportswear or finding a hot spot in the studio to perve on some 'hottie' as they perform a squat or some other asset-bearing exercise. I suppose people are motivated by various factors, and it sometimes can seem as if some individuals purely come to the gym to perve on unexpected candidates. With mobile phone technology encompassing cameras it's easier for predators to snap away at their victims wherever and whenever. An 'innocent' person texting on their mobile phone in the changing rooms can be harmless, or it can be an undercover ploy to take various snapshots of nudity which may be used for their evening's pleasure! It happens, but how can you tell, short of grabbing the phone from the potential violator and checking for yourself! Oops, you're texting your mum – continue!

Regardless of the reason for visiting the gym whether it is to workout or perve, in true Poser Paradise Gyms-style, keeping it cheap and cheery was definitely their model for presumed success within the company. The motto they proclaimed was 'affordable fitness for everyone'. Affordable at what expense though! Holes in the wall that were an emblem of the untrained exerciser, who thought the heavy weight they were lifting was possible, were often covered up with posters or machines. The machines, however, often broke down with members having to wait weeks for a part to be delivered by some faraway country. Why can't the parts ever be manufactured in the UK? That's right, it's a cheaper way of doing it surely. For some members it didn't matter how fully functioning the machines were as in some notorious gyms, it's common to have the workout in the sauna! Well, I guess it can count as part of their three visits to the gym per week!

ATTACK OF THE YOGIS!

In the years I worked at Poser Paradise Gyms and the umpteen yoga sessions I'd taken part in, I had saved up the money to go on a yoga teacher-training course. Having acclimatised myself to the various breeds of member found in a yoga class, I felt now was my time to 'normalise' these creatures to be a little less uptight. My flexibility had improved vastly over the years from less stone-like to more paper! Once qualified, I of course wanted, and got the opportunity, to teach within the club. The yoga teacher who was self-employed at the time and taught a few classes within the club obviously expressed her acknowledgement through her demeanour. Like prey to a predator, she was cautious not to be attacked by my modern approach and interpretation of yoga. Her classes were packed, and as a regular attendee to her class, I had learnt a lot from her. Her name was Linda and it was her class that I experienced my first yogic session with all the various personalities to go with it. I fell in love with yoga for its challenging physical moves more than the spiritual side, and so I taught my classes more with a physical fitness yoga feel to it compared to other styles. As my confidence in teaching grew and my thirst for knowledge broadened into other disciplines like Pilates, I felt my delivery during class sessions was more productive. My class numbers doubled and in some cases trebled to the detriment of Linda's class numbers. I felt bad, but at the same time my ego was being stroked and nurtured and it just felt great. I'd finally found my niche, the thing I loved to do. It comes with the territory, offer a great class to help people and above all keep it 'fresh' and they will come back for more. Was it a case of out with the old, in with the new or two instructors at war, yoga mats to the ready! I attended Linda's class fairly religiously, but when the day came when she came to my class I felt under pressure. Was she coming to check out the competition, learn maybe some new moves or purely to have a workout for herself? Instructors can be very critical about other instructor's classes, and I'm always dubious when an instructor comes to one of my classes as to what their intention is. A few years into teaching group fitness, I started to build my confidence up. It would soon be the case, as I'm sure all instructors experience, that over time with practice and continued learning, when other instructors of the same field attend your class that it wouldn't be such a big deal. The war eventually ended after a year on the battleground. Linda left Poser Paradise Gyms having asked for a pay rise beforehand but literally getting the yoga finger back at her. In fitness, getting a pay rise is as likely as enjoying a session at the dentist getting your wisdom teeth ripped out.

PILATES – A NEW DIRECTION!

The Pilates course was a natural follow-on from the yoga course. It really did give me the tools to understand the body better for myself and for others. Like most courses I've been on, there's always an interesting array of people that enrol. Pilates was no exception with people committing for all kinds of reasons whether it be for themselves, one-to-one clients, a midlife crisis, it's trendy, for the fact it's time off work or for group fitness, like me. I enlisted as my participation in some Pilates classes in the past had helped my back, and I felt the moves would bring something new to my existing knowledge. A mixture of old and young were the learners who came to add to their existing qualifications. The course's prerequisite was anatomy and physiology. As I've seen on other courses, one or two people were so petrified when it came to standing in front of people. I felt myself reminiscing over teaching K.O.B.O again. Luckily this time without the man killers teaching us! Some individuals came on the course to give them ideas for training their clients on a one-to-one basis, and so I felt sorry for them having to teach this to a group. I did benefit from their misfortune, however, as by observing their delivery, I could reflect, contrast and critique how I would come across when asked to demonstrate my piece. Courses are great for sharing ideas and of course meeting like-minded people with their own stories of how they came to be involved in the industry. Most stories start with 'I've always been interested in fitness; I was a competitive athlete a few years ago and then fitness was the natural course to take'. Then there's me – my laziness and lack of exercise forced me to try things the general population don't like doing. I kind of fell into the industry! On every course there's always one idiot or one completely clueless individual whereby you sit and cringe at the questions they ask. This course was no different. Sometimes common sense prevails, but in some cases some people need a separate course on life studies as in how to get one or how to have one! When it comes to pelvic tilting, you either get it or you don't! Those who were intellectually challenged from a physical sense (i.e., mind not connecting with body) looked, when practising the pelvic tilt, a cross between a belly dancer and someone trying to make love in a highly charged way to the surrounding world from a standing position. Literally the whole body thrusting in a distressed way as if one's ass was on fire. Amusing all the same, it was going to take practice to get it right and to think, these were professionals within the fitness industry whom you would expect to have some kind of body awareness. What chance have the rest of the public got in getting this right? Would this be the start of a nightmare, educating people in how to pelvic tilt? Individuals walking around thrusting their pelvis as if starved of sex!

The Pilates course for beginners was so basic that I was lying there half the time thinking when are we going to move. Was it a test to see if we could lie still for long enough! I could feel my attention deficit disorder kicking in. The room was freezing and made me feel like a piece of bacon sitting in a fridge waiting to be moved and cooked. There was a hell of a lot of course work and case studies to do, and after finishing the beginners', I was enthusiastic to learn the intermediate and advanced levels. Would they challenge me more by perhaps moving two legs at one time or startling me into actually waking up from my coma-induced state? Saying that, I can't knock the beginners' as it was definitely a class designed for those who have limited movement or are fresh out of rehab / physio. I knew though in mainstream health clubs that the beginner Pilates would not bring the numbers into classes in a competitive market whereby if the class numbers weren't busy, you'd be axed. We had to teach the beginners' level for six months to a year before we could move onto a higher level.

The intermediate course was a progression from the beginners' as to be expected and was predominantly based around using equipment like the dyna-band (stretchy band thing) and the Swiss ball (round bouncy ball thing). Having spent years in the fitness industry, I didn't really learn much on the course. Not blowing my own trumpet, but I felt the tutor teaching us knew less than what I did, especially when it came to me asking her questions to gain more of an insight and to try and feel as if I was getting more from the course. Her replies to my questions were at times a bit ropey. There's nothing less inspirational when the teacher, who you look up to with admiration for their knowledge that they possess, is not bringing anything new to your table! Was it just another money spinning course to wangle a few more notes from my pocket? At uni, I was bowled over with the knowledge and research my professors shared with us, and for the fact that all the lecturers drove plush cars and had their own books out. Well, I guess the intermediate Pilates course was another piece of paper to say that I'm now qualified to sit on a ball and do things on it.

The advanced course was the icing on the cake, just what I was looking for. A challenge that would keep me interested and therefore would reflect in my teaching to others and keep them interested too. I could see the bigger picture having achieved all three levels. I could cater for group fitness classes and work with all levels with varying options. Although most beginners always seem convinced they're ready for the advanced exercises even though it's obvious they're not. My Pilates teaching and knowledge soon surpassed that of yoga, and so my focus quickly geared towards looking into how to evolve Pilates moves using the Pilates principles. As for teaching a beginners' class the way I was taught on the course – hell no! Unless of course it was to wake up the dead and get them to achieve the ability of opening their eyes.

OFF WITH THE MARIGOLDS!

The fitness industry has evolved over the years, and the role of fitness instructor has dissipated to my relief and fear. I was relieved for the fact having studied over the years to better myself that my role had progressed from master cleaner to personal trainer (PT). Spit-polishing the dumb-bells was becoming a thing of the past and I found myself actually teaching how to use them! Instead of receiving a salary from the gym, they ingeniously changed the role into one where the PT would pay rent to the gym to train their clients. They of course would help us attain clients through their lucrative, cheap half-hour sessions to get members intrigued in personal training. The half-hour sessions were paid for by the member and pocketed by the company with the PT doing the session for the love of fitness and to, fingers crossed, convert them into a paying client. The conversion rate was high where I worked, but every once in a while there were the duds who you knew just wouldn't want to part with their cash for further personal training sessions. There are some individuals who try to always get something for nothing, sapping your energy and draining you of your resources along the way. Sharing knowledge from instructor to member should never be grudged, but there needs to be an equilibrium to what is said and how much is said. Personal training courses, amongst others, can be very expensive and once this knowledge has been acquired it's only fair that PTs reap the rewards from this newfound knowledge when passing it on to others. Saying that, it's kind of taking the piss if you charge for everything. Going to the toilet can be seen as a health and safety issue or a force of nature, but if a member asks where the toilet is, and as a newfound fully fledged PT you say, 'For that information it'll cost you', well, it's not going to build the client base is it! There can be an expectation from members for PTs to quickly write them a personalised programme for free with little understanding to the complexity and time involved in writing one. Having joined the gym, members feel an entitlement to get a programme written for them not fully understanding that many PTs in gyms are self-employed, and like the members, the PTs are also paying for the privilege to be there.

The obvious fear of no longer being employed was having to pay the club a rental regardless if people converted to personal training or not. All the trainers were apprehensive. Would the members in the local area pay for one to-one training? It would make or break the strong from the weak. The better the salesperson, the more chance of making a success at PT regardless of how shit the PT was at instructing. When I was there, all the PTs were pretty good. David, a fellow PT and good mate of mine, often thought the quieter PTs within the team would struggle, purely for the fact they weren't salespeople. How would they be able to sell themselves as a product to others? Would they find their nerve to approach people to persuade them to part with their cash? Could they personify a 'you need me' kind of attitude? Surprisingly, all things turned out pretty damn good. There were those PTs who had the gift of the gab, those who fluttered their long, pretty eyelashes to the opposite sex or in some cases (and cleverly) the same sex and of course those who knew their fitness knowledge inside out. In what was to become a more competitive field, new strategies were adopted in order to avoid drowning in the deep end. Tactics would be deployed in whatever form they had to in order to attract new or keep existing clientele! At first, it seemed as if the new PT product would simply and solely benefit the health clubs. It did in fact build us into stronger, competitive independent PTs and would pave the way for the survival of the fittest. Had we finally escaped the realms of 'Just Over Broke' (aka JOB) and the marigolds?

Over time, personal training has exploded throughout the fitness industry with many other fitness organisations clambering onboard. It's not just for the rich and famous, Poser Paradise Gyms made it accessible for everyone, which in turn transformed the fitness industry into a personal training culture full of the kind and caring, the egotistical, to the complete moron!

CHAPTER THREE

LONDON – TIME TO UP THE ANTICS!

Poser Paradise Gyms was a great stepping stone in my fitness career. It gave me the necessities to survive the industry and for the challenges to come. I lasted longer than I did at Relish Fitness. Three years was pretty good going but as things felt a little stale and more like a prison sentence, it was time to move. My marigolds had quickly thinned, and so a decision had to be made. Buy new ones or leave! So I left for the big smoke. London with all that it offers: an abundance of health clubs, opportunities, more people with more needs, and with these needs came extra challenges – mentally, physically and emotionally!

I moved to a rented place in Surrey Quays, which was near enough to the city centre for work. The rent was twice as expensive as my mortgage back up in Scotland and the house smelt of cat piss! I suppose if you pay cheap, you get cheap. It was an excuse to spend longer at work and to build up my PT business. I managed to get a transfer from the Dundee club to one based just off The Strand and joined the team as a full-time PT. There are many gyms in London with some literally next door to each other. Some are like matchboxes trapped literally six feet under! Perhaps an insight into the austerity that these gyms can hold for both members and staff! No natural light, smells of sewage and sweat, with loud music and uninterested staff in a place full of gym politics were just part of the perks for joining up. Getting dressed in the changing room was like changing in a small cupboard. One minute you're tying your shoelaces, and then as soon as you stand upright, the lights go out! It's at this point you realise your head has disappeared up someone's ass! Not bad going for my first time in London – a home with a strong odour of cat piss and a work life underground, in a matchbox and smelling of vinegar. Apart from this, I was mesmerised. Everything was new and exciting with the opportunities that could be possible within the city. I was on a sliding scale whereby I didn't pay any gym rent for the first month to allow me to build up my clientele. PT courses, I guess, like any course, fuel you to believe the impossible. People need trainers true, but is it as simple as approaching a person and making them understand the benefits of training with you? Hell, no! So many people, aka the gym regulars, suffer from body dysmorphia. Approaching paranoid Annie can turn out to be an hour of explaining to her that, 'No, you don't look as if you need help, I just thought that I could offer you some help'. I gave up with my body dysmorphia after two years of trying to put on weight in the form of muscle. My trainer, when I first started out in the world of fitness, inspired me but at the same time gave me a complex to how small my frame was in comparison to his. Whether it's a case of self-awareness or the culture of the gym, which places an imposition of how you should look, is something I'm still working out!

OK, looking like the Hulk would not suit me and having a bigger chest than my mother would just look weird but just a little extra size would've been nice. There is a competitive nature within the gym environment from the changing room to the gym floor. Disillusioned paranoia suffered by many, including myself, can occur simply by the pretence of the gym surroundings. There's a generalised understanding that achieving 'the perfect body' requires some work. The first-timer to the more advanced exerciser all strive for it! It's only when starting a regime for ultimate results that 'a workout' turns into virtually rupturing your lungs to the point of wobbling out of the gym looking for the nearest accident and emergency (A & E). Achieving a ripped body is something which requires a life change. This involves losing all sense of life and making the gym your home, your body your temple and as for friends, well, thank God for Facebook. I'll update you with my life through there. Some people can easily train twice a day and others can look upon these people with a slight admiration and a desire to be like them (or is it bewilderment and a sense of 'get a life'). This is where the disillusion part kicks in. Not knowing that some people make the gym their life, and as a result, yes, their bodies are looking mighty fine, but it's impossible to achieve if you only attend the gym twice a week! Every so often during a training session, the audience get a sneak preview at the 'body beautiful' who at regular intervals look in the mirror, lift their vest to expose and tease the rest of the mere mortals in the gym that they have a long way to go. Even if the 'body beautiful' are training their legs, there's an impulsiveness to check the six-pack to see if it's still there, or perhaps it's the exhibitionist within themselves showing the rest of us their personalities. It could be a commendation to oneself, a kind of self-appraisal. 'Well done me for looking so wonderful!'

Walking around the gym looking for potential clients can be like a lion to its prey. Not necessarily scouring for victims to pounce on but acknowledging those who can really use some attention. There are those who walk on the treadmill slowly and cautiously as if walking the tight rope or having shat their pants. Apart from taking up treadmill space, wouldn't they benefit from not paying a membership and to just go for regular walks around the park? Week in, week out, the same treadmill is used by the same person, going at the same speed, for the same time. A feeling of achievement is felt by the user for the simple fact that they have attended the gym, but is there not a feeling of frustration for not seeing any changes in their body? It's not easy for PTs to approach these individuals to offer them advice, i.e., point where the increase button is for the speed or the incline. Unfortunately, gyms have mirrors and the preyed upon can see the predator creeping towards the treadmill. A force field builds around them with the growing self-acknowledgment of 'I know what I'm doing; I've been doing this treadmill walk for months. I will not pay for any form of advice'. The gym goers, like retail shoppers, have the same mental attitude that the customer is always right – who the fuck made up that rule!

So the search for clients is a psychologist's wet dream. Days and weeks of assessing the gym member to understand their wants, needs, psychological trauma and other ailments are conducted in order to connect with them and bring them onboard as a client. There are those who are keen to be trained but have hesitation when it comes to paying for it, and there are others, who when spoken to, gesture with a strange look as if it was asked, 'How do you say motherfucker in French!'

In London, a month passes very quickly. The second month would see me paying a reduced rate for using the gym and then by the third month I would be paying the full rate of £700, which today is phenomenally cheap for London. That's a lot of psychological evaluation. Building a client base wasn't easy, and with my passion lying within the studio, I decided to increase my group fitness teaching to take the pressure off from the burden of more bills to pay. I was freelance and at times felt like a prostitute to fitness, walking the streets looking for gyms that would want to take me on as a group fitness professional proving that, yes, I can bend over and touch my toes for a fee! I offered to do free sessions to get my foot in the door. As the offers to teach one or two classes came by consequence of my hard grafting, so did the opportunity to do a group fitness manager role. It would be the opportunity to become a manager and avoid paying the full rental at the gym where I did personal training. It would be a time-out card from trawling through the gym for potential clients, which often felt like a glorified salesman wandering around a modern mental asylum picking those who didn't seem too disturbed with life's dramas and torment to buy into your service! Then again, the more disturbed could really do with the distraction from their lives and their minds and utilise a trainer to offload their unwanted baggage and stress! I often ended up with the latter!

I laugh now as many people who enter the industry have this conception that clients will happen at the click of a finger, not realising it takes hard grafting of many hours of non-paid work to sometimes get just one or two clients. Having a degree in psychology had its uses! A handful of clients who come twice a week for a one-to-one session will perhaps clear the gym rent for the month. There's then the challenge to find the clients who will help fund the cost for you living in the city. London is such a transient place whereby people get their fix, make their money and leave within the space of five to ten years to raise a family or to breathe fresh air and drink clean water! Keeping people on your books is a constant testament of time and energy. New faces require new approaches, as one strategy to get someone enrolled doesn't necessarily work the same for everyone!

New fitness consultants who roam around the gym floor look clueless and dazed with what to do. The lack of guidance from their peers can be the rise or fall of their future PT career. The lack of interpersonal skills they possess can also be their downfall. Unfortunately, personality and how to have one aren't taught on the gym courses they attend. Then again, some only attend these courses as a means to continue receiving their Jobseeker's Allowance! They have no passion to help people, but they simply have their eyes on the prize – pounds per hour instead of having personality with people! Within each club there can be anything from five to thirty five PTs advertised on the club boards. Whether you ever see most of them in the gym is a different matter. Profile boards bunched together on the wall display a mug shot of the PT and their credentials! In some cases it can all rather look like some portfolio from some dating site! 'Pick me' etched all over the advert with some of them posing and flexing muscles that should simply be covered up or used in some form of porn magazine! Desperation isn't an admirable quality, and to feel that exposing parts of the body, mainly the torso, is an appeal to the masses is a wrongful conviction! The culture of gym and its imposition through others of 'body beautiful' creep in to those who have interpreted their course, as the only way to be, is to have some form of sculpted egotism.

Over the years, recessions, economic crises and the like have forced PTs to become more cut-throat in business tactics towards their competitors. Newcomers to the industry either have to step up to the mark or waste the thousands of pounds they've spent on their personal training courses to find another job that will start paying their bills. A huge plus factor in the world of personal training is trying to get your identity out there! The best way to connect with others is by taking group fitness classes, either teaching or taking part in them. Walking around the gym floor is often met with resistance and retorts of, 'I know what I'm doing!' Classes can promote your personality and get people talking. Before you know it, your name is around the gym, hopefully on a good note, and the workload then follows! People connect with charisma, not crafty sales talk. Walking around some gyms, I see on the notice boards posters desperately advertising weight loss by some of the PTs. It's a beacon of hope for the avid cake adorer. There often is a 'before and after' shot, which by comparing the two pictures makes you wonder whether picture one is just simply someone pushing out their belly saying, 'Wow, look how pregnant I am and I'm not even pregnant!' This was the case with one PT who did a 'before and after' shot of himself. It was kind of obvious because even though the 'after' picture showed his belly sucked in, it's always difficult pulling in a double chin. Work with this trainer and you'll shed the pounds! Another known case was where the PT hadn't shaved or washed his hair for several days, ate literally a large four course meal to bloat himself and then took his 'before' picture to show him at his worst. The 'after' shot picture, of course, had him clean-shaven, hair washed and styled, spray tanned to give the healthy-glow look, and before the picture could be taken, a quick set of press ups and arm curls to pump up his upper body. His posture, of course, was miraculously 'Pilatesque' – upright and proud with the final icing on the cake – 'the smile' of how great life is now! What the poster fails to tell the reader is that in order to lose the weight you need to train around three to four times a week which either means you fork out four times the hourly rate the PT is charging, or if you're skint train with them once a week and come to the gym another two or three times within the week! Now, the chances are if someone is overweight, it's because potentially, not always the case, they like their food and hate to exercise! To expect someone to come into the gym on their own accord, unless super motivated to shed the pounds, is setting someone up for failure! The intelligent PTs will get their clientele to participate in 'worthy' group fitness classes along with their one-to-one training sessions. This will get their client into the gym more often and allows more than just the PT to crack the whip to help them achieve their goals. If results are seen by the person trying to achieve them, then it's a win-win situation for both PT and client! Some PTs have still to learn this phenomena.

TIME TO MANAGE!

The studio role was a chance to manage a group of fellow instructors. It was something different, something fresh and something that would feel similar to placing chopsticks under my nostrils and slamming my head down hard. Imagine Maria Carey working for you and the demands that would follow. OK, most instructors didn't want their own dressing room before class performance or fresh flowers delivered to the studio before class, but sometimes the expectations of some would supersede what the individual clubs could actually deliver. Most fitness clubs are so restricted with their budgets that it's a constant fight to fix the stereo, replace the head microphone or mats or pay good instructors the rate that they deserve! Budget and business can work together, but when it's to the detriment of losing good instructors, which in turn loses paying members, the club has a problem. I've been to many condescending meetings where the guys in charge project and forecast their findings of how they can close the backdoor to stop members leaving their gyms. Short of putting a gun to people's head exclaiming leave and I'll shoot. It's a gym; gyms aren't exactly the majority of people's favourite choice. Changing attitudes towards the gym are hardly going to change much. There isn't going to be a mass orgy of people fighting their way into the gym anytime soon because they've had trouble sleeping with the thought of missing out on running on the treadmill. Time and time again, I hear ideas and efforts to retain members by offering a better service, a better product or ways to incentivise staff by 'glamming' up some shitty bonus structure that would give them the opportunity to perhaps buy a latte at the end of the month. It's true of the saying – pay peanuts, get monkeys, and boy, there are many monkeys in many gyms. Motivation and morale for the salespeople, member service and reception team tend to be low as the goal posts or gym politics constantly change as new ideas are simply regurgitated under a different format. The gyms expect a lot from their staff but give so little in return or in some cases a free water bottle and the chance to workout in the gym for free, whoopee! Turnover tends to be incredibly high as there are only so many peanuts one can eat before the realisation settles in that bills need to be paid. The sales team can be paid a ball-crunching, penny-pinching salary of around twelve to eighteen thousand pounds per year with the possibility to top up their income through commission! How can they survive in an expensive place like London! Perhaps selling bags of cocaine at a profitable price for those keen to lose weight the quick way! Oh, hold on, that has happened! As the goal posts for commission constantly change for the sales team making it harder and harder to reach their targets, methods are adopted to 'make the money!' This can take many forms! In one club, which was mentioned in a Watchdog documentary and where a good mate of mine was the manager at the time, the sales team would get people to sign contracts without allowing the potential members time to read what they were signing! In some cases signatures were fraudulently used especially when it was the end of the month and targets had to be met and bonuses had to be collected! In this particular club, new members signed up with a belief from the sales guy that a brand new state of the art swimming pool was going to be built over the next few months! Of course, no swimming pool had even passed the planning stage, and as for the sales person, well, once the commission was received it was time to abandon ship before suspicion grew! From one ship to another, the salesperson would simply get transferred to another club or company, which was potentially opening their brand new state of the art swimming pool too! As for me, the salespeople made managing group fitness tougher.

Manipulative sales tactics would get new potential members to take part in classes for free with a belief that brand new classes and more classes were going to be introduced to the timetable, just to bag the sale! If a potential member was looking for a particular style of class not advertised on the timetable, of course this would be launching soon! Once enrolled, the new members would then tap at my doorstep wondering why the extra additions were not being introduced to the timetable.

The longevity for Poser Paradise Gyms is questionable as they continue to haemorrhage out money on ridiculous ideas and concepts without consulting those on the shop floor. After all, poor management equals piss-poor performance! Virtually all the ideas that I've seen introduced have nosedived into the depths of 'what the fuck', as they are never followed up with proper training or advertising. The PTs, instructors, salespeople, member service and reception team all see it first hand and they understand the wants and needs of the members, not those stuck in offices all day, brainstorming ideas of how to appease the shareholders and shaft everybody at the same point. So when it comes to ordering new mats and new stereos for the instructors, it's a waiting game, a long waiting game.

How does the gym close the back door? Group fitness, invest in group fitness! It's where the heart and soul of the gym is, a party atmosphere driven by a great instructor, a place where people can share the monotony and drudgery of exercise together. Where are all the great instructors? Well, they tend to be found in places that appreciate them for what they deliver and how they deliver it in the form of payment. Some fitness companies have reduced (and some continue to do so) the rates of pay for their instructors for whatever bullshit reason they give. As always, group fitness professionals receive normally a quarterly letter (in some cases, daily) from the studio manager. It goes something like;

Hey guys
I just want to thank you all for your hard work and for keeping your classes busy to a high standard (note; letters always start with positive psychology to give the reader hope).

Due to the club receiving its new budget for the year (note; here comes the bad news), some classes will need to be removed from the timetable (note; shit, I knew I should've bought the studio manager chocolates on a regular basis – I hope it's not my class even though it's busy). A new rate of pay has been revised and the hourly rate per class will be £5 less than what you're getting (note; obviously making sure there's an even shafting for everyone across the board). I understand if you are not happy with this change (note; no shit, Sherlock, I'm absolutely delighted, what makes you think I'm pissed off) then please give me two weeks' notice if you want to give up your class! (note; taught here for eight years with no pay rise and now the rate's getting dropped, of course I'm going to give my loyalty through thick and thin).

On a separate note, instructors are required to bring their own batteries for the head microphone (note; batteries are expensive), a head microphone belt (note; another expense) and make sure you turn up ten minutes before your class too! (note; obviously ten minutes of not getting paid).

If you have any questions (note; why are you so good to me?) please don't hesitate to contact myself in the club.

Keep up the hard work (note; we will for less money, no problems) and have a great day (note; well it was great up until reading this letter – can't wait for the next edition).

I found myself as studio manager writing these bullshit letters and want to apologise to everyone I inflicted this pain and torment on! It's hard to swallow the reduction especially when members' rates and PT rent increase. The hardest thing is the fact we motivate others with what we do, and we are expected to motivate others by those who employ us, however, who motivates us? Oh, that's right, we're in the industry for the passion of fitness. OK, in that case then give my income to some charity. I can restrict my diet to bread, water and peanuts, walk everywhere and I can also tell those I'm due money to, i.e., the Inland Revenue that I'm not paying my way because I'm passionate about what I do! They'll just have to understand. Some instructors in the industry annoyingly and casually use the 'passion' reason for being in the industry, and I guess they are humbled souls that have another source of income through some other means.

At the end of the day, passion does not always equal knowledge and competence, so therefore there's the frustration of those who get paid because they are passionate about what they do, and then there are those who have passion with unsurpassable knowledge and competency who get the same rate. Is it the case that some of those individuals who are passionate about their fitness careers just lack that little touch of technical capability or perhaps it's self-acceptance for what they're worth. I remember a fairly new instructor two years into teaching whinging to me, as we like to do from time to time, about the fact she'd never had a pay increase, and how she felt she was worth more. Little did she realise I'd been teaching for around ten years and had rarely seen any form of increase apart from foreigners attending classes who couldn't understand the language, but I didn't want to ruin her day altogether, so kept silent. I've seen the same girl in question teach her Pilates class and as many instructors do – analyse; I identified her technique as unique! Her plank position looked as if her lower spine had collapsed making her belly hang out like some beer-bellied man crawling across the bar floor for his next pint! She wants a pay rise! I guess it's a belief in her passion that she deserves one, or perhaps the only rise she should be focusing on is her hips and belly!

A slimeball of a general manager decided in one club to reduce everyone's class rate. He removed a couple of classes, one being mine, in order to bring in one or two of his own mates. The rate reduction was presumed for cutting costs and adhering to strict budgets; however, it helped to pay the manager and his mates the higher of the rates offered to freelance instructors. This unfortunately is common practice. Karma did eventually bite him in the ass, and he was fired to the delight of many!

As a group fitness manager, there was the daily hassle and regular complaints of equipment that didn't work. A stereo that crackles or craps out during a song can be highly frustrating for the professional trying to conduct the class. I know I've experienced this many times, and members look at you as if it's your fault. The class ends up being shit, instructor morale goes down and then they, both instructor and members, approach me, the group fitness manager, as to when the stereo will get fixed. How long's a piece of string? If only they knew I was on a shoestring budget for all things studio related and to order anything new would result in filling an encyclopaedia worth of order forms. Bring in your own stereo or multitask by singing and instructing at the same time! Group fitness manager was a thankless task. There were no funds for new projects or investing in quality instructors and this is generally the same across the board. There were the issues of instructors who weren't professional enough to find their own cover while away on holiday and subsequently no one would show up for the class. A barrage of unhappy members for not getting their daily dose of fitness would queue up to stab the man in charge, ME!

With all studio timetables there follows the daunting task of axing classes that just don't fill the studio. Having to explain to the instructor can be a horrible process. Having to explain to the members why their class is being removed can be a case of life and death and can pave the way for a new season of CSI! In one club, the manager had given me the joyous task of reducing the expenditure of the class timetable, which meant either reducing the rate of pay to instructors in order to keep the timetable filled with classes or dropping the least popular classes. The kickboxing class within this club was consistently quiet pulling in a handful of dedicated people per week. I explained to the instructor, low numbers and cutting back as reasons for removing his class, and he then reiterated this back to his members. I had a knock on the office door with the instructor on the other end asking me to come into the studio and face the angry members. I understand members' frustration losing a class, but when they sign a contract for the gym it does state class timetables will change from season to season. Besides, I thought to myself, if you pay cheap membership, expect cheap service! Some instructors, at this point of removing their class, see it as a personal attack on them, and it can be the case, however, it should be expected in an environment that is numbers focused. Quiet classes equal 'see ya later!'

Entering the studio, the discussion began and ended up becoming an influx of insults and attacks. One member somehow managed to get onto the subject of how successful he was and how he was richer than me! I looked on with disbelief and calmly stated that if money wasn't an issue, then perhaps the class could be a pay class where members pay for the privilege for utilising the studio. By this time, in my mind, my middle finger was fully extended craving to turn to the arrogant guy and say 'fuck you'. I'm simply doing a job and explained to everybody concerned that another class could replace the kickboxing with the hopeful intention of satisfying more members. I really wanted to say, 'Look you're a member of Poser Paradise Gyms, what the hell do you expect!' Trying to reason with unreasonable people though made the task more arduous. The class was removed and my head was still firmly intact. The general manager received a handful of complaints from the kickboxing crew in the coming weeks, and as a result he quickly reinstated the class back on the timetable. Undermining my position, the manager made me look like a complete joke for removing the class in the first place. Was he a wimp of a manager or did he have two fingers firmly pressed against his asshole? I wanted to say to the members, 'Hey, it's this idiot manager who wanted to cut the timetable down and agreed with me that the kickboxing class had to go because of low attendance.' So the manager gets the pat on the back for saving the day, and I'm the one who receives the evil stares and gets pelted with rotten eggs as I walk through the gym. Well, not quite rotten eggs but the looks did stink!

The toughest part about freelancing and managing the studio is that it's all about capacity! If the demand isn't there, neither will the class be before long! Maybe when I'm teaching my classes in future, I should carry some cardboard cut-outs of people to scatter throughout the studio and dim the lights to create the image of yet another busy class! The film 'Home Alone' springs to mind. Consistently busy classes are not possible by anybody's standards!

Strangely enough, I served my sentence in this job role managing group fitness for different clubs for about eight years. It was great for securing some kind of income but ended up making me feel like I was some call-centre complaints hotline and purely someone to pass the buck on to. Never again! It's difficult to manage and make changes to freelancers' schedules and finances. I myself was a freelancer in other clubs experiencing the same shit I was expected to dish out through my role! Different clubs in London have different issues in regards to the studio. Depending on where in London you are will depend on the clientele that utilise the studio classes. The snobs, the wannabes, the ghetto dwellers, the confrontational, the simplistic, the demanding, the hard workers to those who really do need a dumb-bell shoved up their ass to do something are just a select few who frequent certain studios. I've managed group fitness in all corners of London. Some clubs are distinctly hard working, Shepherds Bush is full of Aussies and South Africans and they certainly love to punish themselves to extreme fitness. Central London clubs have the businessmen and women, who, and I know from working with some of them, are only able to lift as much as what their laptop weighs. Saying that there are quite a few who are buffed and toned in the central clubs, so I can't be too harsh and stereotype all business people. One club sticks in my mind like chewing gum to the shoe! The ghetto club of Walworth road, South London! With locker doors hanging off the hinges and cracked windows in every pane of glass, it gave an unsettling feeling just on the approach to the gym with what felt like some Eminem music video. I had taken over the studio on a part-time basis just helping out and decided to increase the classes on the timetable to give the club a greater boost on all levels. Standing back at first and looking into the studio to watch the classes in their prime made me gasp in horror at the shockingly poor level of the instructors.

Everything was wrong about the studio from the instructors' unmotivated stances, their prehistoric teaching, to the general attitude of the class itself! Instructors who have taught in a club for many years can easily fall into the dilemma of safety and comfort! There's a deluded belief that years of experience count in the fitness industry and with it follows a general lapse to re-educate oneself or update one's knowledge within an evolving business! The style of training was archaic to say the least, and speaking to these 'unwilling to change, it's always been like this'-type instructors was a mission impossible! It was a gym that seemed to date back to the 'Jane Fonda' era of leggings and lycra! Even the weights looked as if they were made from sculpted rock from a pre-dinosaur era! One female instructor, who was obviously very popular, had about sixty people crammed into a studio that could hold thirty. Perhaps slightly excusable if it was a class to train people in how to stand on a crowded bus, but no, it was an aerobics class with hand weights. A recipe for disaster! Swinging weights while prancing around made me cringe in horror. Where on earth did she learn 'or read' to teach like that? I praised her for her popular class but explained that maximum capacity was thirty people. A busy class doesn't necessarily mean an effective class! How can sixty people move freely in a space for thirty? Besides, lack of variety on a timetable can force people into the one class, or perhaps a popular class is down to a 'lovely' instructor teaching it. I've been smacked in the face twice in that class but she's such a lovely instructor, that's why I go'.

Dropping a hectic class to one that was more manageable seemed to cause a problem for what I can only imagine was her ego being punctured! Before long, arguments were exchanged between both myself and the instructor to a level whereby I had to axe her from the club for the simple fact she was a freelancer not willing to adhere to club policies! Like a red rag to a bull, a few days after replacing her, she came into the club with her supposed lawyer to prove a case of unfair dismissal. Shocked but intrigued at the same time, I asked this so-called lawyer for her business card and proof that she was who she was, and to no surprise, she failed to comply. Perhaps a friend who liked the idea of acting like a lawyer for the axed instructor who was actually illegally on the premises; after all the dismissal letter did state to not enter the particular club while dismissed! After weeks of constant issues within the club and a fear that I would get lynched when leaving the gym at night, I decided to give up the studio in that particular club. It wasn't worth the hassle and the lack of appreciation I was given for trying to improve and enhance the club, and besides, I didn't fancy myself as a 'Jack Bauer' stand-in for '24 season 9'!

The role of group fitness manager was sometimes altered to Studio and Events Manager or SEM for short. SEM made me feel like I was back in my SRO days; it just covered up the fact I had to deal with people's shit on a daily basis. The events side of it normally consisted of finding ways to create things without any expense: putting on a master class with perhaps two instructors teaching it but at the cost of one instructor; supplying ice lollies before, during and after classes; offering a discount on sun beds which did piss off Monika, a black lady, who said it wasn't fair on black people as what use would sun beds be to them. I know Monika well and replied to her with, 'You're lucky you don't need to waste your money on sun beds to get colour!' She laughed, but it was a fair point from her so we threw in a chance to win a beauty therapy session for everybody to benefit from. Happy people all round.

Unfortunately there has been for donkey years a consistent rate paid out to all instructors for classes taught. Regardless of whether teaching for one year or twenty-one years, how skilled or experienced one is, how many members one attracts to a class or any other factor, the rate is the same for everyone. When first starting in group fitness it can be exciting and pretty good money. As the years tick by however, and the experience and knowledge grows, the money unfortunately doesn't. For those who play it right, it can be very fruitful, paying dividends. For those who accept the rate and continue to whinge about the lack of appreciation they get are destined to continue to dispel the rate by saying, 'I teach for the passion of fitness'. Obviously they live with their parents! In terms of the fitness industry, those who opt for the freelance route can prove very lucrative for them if choosing the correct location and company. They can set up their own company or have other strategies to market themselves as a product. Everybody for themselves! I too have passion for what I do and that's group fitness; however, there comes a time where I fancy some of the good things in life not just the ability to afford coffee with cake!

CHAPTER FOUR

IT'S A CLASS ACT!

Being enclosed inside the studio away from the outside world and management was pure escapism. Not being told what to do and having control over what to do spurred my creative side. Of course, and similar to outside in the gym, the studio can have its own unique environment. The introverts, extroverts, workers, non-workers, married, singletons, fit, non-fit, psychologically disturbed, mentally deranged to the physically challenged are a select few of the candidates that the group fitness professional has to contend with on a normal day.

Being motivated comes naturally for most instructors but it can be a highly draining experience with just the simplest of tasks like approaching the studio door. Outside there can stand an abundance of group exercisers eager to gain entry into the studio for their class fix. Before arriving at the gates to the studio (aka the doors), and before I even get the chance to smile to everyone there are always a few complainers eager to highlight the fact the class inside the studio is running a minute late. Some go as far as explaining in detail the problems that arise in the club, like the toilet being out of order for months or classes which have been cancelled. I don't give two flying fucks but I can't exactly say that to a member, it's not politically correct although very tempting just to see their reaction! Instead I tilt my head to one side with a sympathetic look as if to say wow, this club is really going downhill. I often wish at times like this that I had a leaflet for 'feed the starving children of Africa' to bring some perspective to the situation!

Class cancellations in some members' eyes are like saying there's a death in the family, it's just unacceptable regardless of how inevitable it can be. How could an instructor abandon their people in their moment of need? How selfish! It's an unfortunate but true part of life that instructors are human too and do from time to time fall ill and need time off. Illness can be sudden and therefore class cancellations are an eventuality. Most instructors are freelance and rely on their income from the classes so most will endeavour to teach the class if they can still stand on two feet without projecting vomit like the girl from 'The Exorcist'. I'm not often ill but when I have been, on my return to teach the class, it's often met with a police-style interrogation as to why I wasn't teaching the week before. Following the interrogation, there is the breakdown analysis of how shit the cover instructor was, or in some cases the cover may have just passed the expectations from some of the tougher judges. The life of an instructor is a constant performance! You're only as good as your last class, and there are always others keen to step in your shoes. If a fellow instructor happens to be very chummy with the group fitness manager, GAME OVER! It's only a matter of time before the group fitness manager will find a reason to change the class or axe it altogether to accommodate their buddy or themselves onto the timetable. If you're extra special in the eyes of the group fitness manager, you may be lucky to bag two classes back to back. I say, if you can't beat them, join them by sending text messages to the person in charge – 'you're such a great instructor, you should be a presenter' or by mentioning some other positive, superficial ego-altering comment to remain in the good books of the person running the show! If you don't, someone else will!

When inside the studio it can sometimes take ten minutes to actually start the class depending on what club it is and how the previous class has left the studio. If the class prior to mine is an aerobics style class, it's guaranteed that the studio will be cold. The more arctic the conditions, the greater the volume of complaints! In some clubs the demands from members run so high that it feels like the members run the club. Instructors from a previous class have literally been threatened by members to put the heating on ten minutes before the end of their class so the next class has a more pleasing environment. It's a gym for crying out loud! We're not there to be happy!

Those needing counselling will tend to approach me at the start of the class to list either their ailments or their psychological disturbances. Some people have a string of conditions larger than a medical dictionary. Whether it is the case or perhaps a psychological prognosis of a slight touch of hypochondria, who knows. I remember when I studied psychology, by the end of my degree I had self-diagnosed myself with about twenty-one conditions stemming from obsessive-compulsive-disorder (OCD) to seasonal affective disorder (SAD) so I know it's easy to be persuaded with the things we read! In some cases I need to cut off the flow of conversation during some counselling sessions as it can take a long time to listen to the issues raised. By this time, there's often a class full of people on the mat listening into the whole conversation, which can stem from irritable bowel syndrome (IBS) to divorcing the husband. Once I've dropped off my bag and put the heating and the CD on, I then float through the class to find out if there are any newcomers or injuries. As I stroll through the mass of people I hope along the way I don't get someone's life story as interesting as it can be. Time is ticking and there are some who glare at the clock, then turn to stare at me with a look as if to say when are you going to start the class! Voila, ten minutes gone! Sometimes I feel like the Jerry Springer to Pilates – a lot of chat, a lot of bitching and within some clubs, arguments exchanged between members. I've still yet to witness mat throwing, strap whipping and block bashing! On my tour around the class there can be many things brought to my attention as I begin to instruct. Looking around the room at the variety of people can help gauge the level the participants are at and can prepare you for what kind of session is about to be encountered. In some instances it can be easily identified who are the first-timers in comparison to the frequent exercisers, not just by how they move but also by how they dress. Wardrobe malfunction during exercise is common, and from the front row position that an instructor has, it can be an eyeful. Bending and twisting can push and pull parts of the body all over the place and in some cases, push things out from their home location. Before you know it, there can be an eye-to-eye confrontation, which is often unknown to the participant. What to do? What to say? Short of saying 'put the mouse back in the house' to the embarrassment of the exerciser, or perhaps plan the next move with a little more thought taking into consideration people's attire. The latter is always the preferred option and is a lesson for the instructor for future classes to take note of people's dress sense at the start of the class and to plan ahead. It's not always members who suffer at the hands of 'wardrobe malfunction'! A mate of mine, also an instructor, was teaching her Body Pump class. She was pumping away doing a tricep kickback whilst on all fours when, unknown to her, her breast popped out. It took a few seconds for her to notice it but when the realisation kicked in she professionally styled it out by declaring she would show both breasts the following week. Fortunately for her, the guy she fancied was in the very front row. Was he thinking 'Wow, I wish I was pumping more than this dumb-bell'? He didn't return to the class the following week! Honestly, what does it take to keep members happy in class?

At the start of every class, I always ask the group if there are any injuries or pregnancies and nine times out of ten nobody will divulge if they do. Some people like to keep their injuries private and some want to challenge you as an instructor to see how good you are at guessing the condition. Listening is definitely an art form that can be a class in itself. Some people simply do not listen to simple instructions, and as a result there can be several people copying everything I do. From scratching my head to itching my ass, yes, it would all be mimicked by those who just copy actions, not words. Even whilst demonstrating different levels of an exercise (beginners', intermediate or advanced) some people will simply work through all the options to my amusement and sometimes frustration (depending on my mood).

THE PREGNANT WOMAN!

I had a pregnant woman who for some reason felt the need to not tell me she was pregnant at the beginning of a Pilate's class. In some women it can be obvious that they are pregnant, others manage to hide it well. It can be a delicate area as I found out during one class I taught. Having asked the injury / pregnancy question, I began the class. I noticed a girl with a bump around the belly area. Thinking to myself, she looks slim all over, it's just her belly that has the bulge. If she is pregnant then she should be doing other options. I approached her during an exercise and crouched down to advise her to take the easier option. She frustratingly turned around and snapped, 'I'm not pregnant, the yoga teacher asked me this as well!' Quickly I responded with, 'No, I didn't ask if you were pregnant, did you not say you had a spinal injury to me last week?' Even though I knew she had never been to my class before.

Play dumb, play ignorant and phew, she replies with a calmer, 'No, I wasn't here last week!'

To make it sound convincing, I asked curiously again, 'Are you sure you weren't here last week, I must be thinking of someone else?' I then started to creep back away from the wounded victim having insulted her on many levels. Embarrassed for both her and myself, I continued with the rest of the class. I never saw her again!

The woman who was actually pregnant and concealed her pregnancy came up to me at the end of the class and said, 'Thanks for the class, by the way I'm four months pregnant!'

By this time I wanted to reply with, 'You WERE pregnant! After the back flips, twisting and crunching I think there's a high probability that you can save your money on buying baby clothes. I think somewhere between the crunch with twist and the taking your legs over your head part was where the decision was made for you of whether a baby was happening or not!' Although in reality I can only recommend that next time choose the options that work for you without feeling obliged to copy the person next to you, and in future TELL any potential group fitness professional of your pregnancy. Political correctness – how annoying! Having spoken to fellow instructors, depending on their mood especially if they are having an off day, when a pregnant woman walks into class, there can be a sigh and the thought of, could you not go to someone else's class. I understand this dilemma, and it's the wrong thought process I know, but especially in a beginners' class I've seen men choosing the pregnancy option getting confused with the various options to one exercise. 'Are you pregnant?' I'll sarcastically ask the guy performing the exercise! The art of listening creeps in yet again. If people listened, then pregnant women wouldn't pose such a great issue. Not that I personally find it an issue but can understand the frustration of others with those fitness programmes, which are pre-choreographed. Some routines don't give the space through timing of a move to list options. Some pre-choreographed classes don't give the necessary information to the 'lazy learning' instructor and therefore there's a sense of having to think for oneself if the 'pregnancy dilemma' arises! Some clubs offer pregnancy classes, and ideally if all clubs offered the same thing, class life would be a little less stressful for some members and the 'lazy' instructor! However budgets prevail and pregnancy classes aren't feasible to penny-pinching gyms.

THE INJURED!

A classic and recurring situation is normally discovered at the end of the class. There's always the odd one, normally two (i.e., the pregnant one), that hang around to confess that they've had an injury, and it's normally something along the lines of having been involved in a serious accident a few weeks ago, spine broken in twenty places and then pose the question, 'Pilates is all right isn't it?' As if trying to convince themselves that what they have just done is absolutely fine. Well, actually no, you've just made your back a hell of a lot worse, and now I recommend, if you're listening, to go straight to the hospital as you're probably going to collapse with the shock and stress inflicted on your body. Enjoy the weekend! Sometimes at the end of the class I feel the need to not just thank the members for coming to the class, but thank myself for enduring a session of sometimes non-listeners, injury prone to the injured silent!

THE FIRST-TIMER!

Apart from not mentioning injuries or pregnancies, the first-time exerciser is often in a world of their own and avoid, or hate admitting, it's their first time. Most of the time they rock up to class late, like some diva celebrity, not understanding the concept of a warm-up – reduce injuries and prepare the body for what's to come. Why is it first-timers are virtually always late for class? Are they trying to work out how to close the lockers, do they get lost en route from changing room to studio or do they stand outside the door waiting for it to be answered by the instructor and then finally realise they should just walk in? If they have an injury or are pregnant, do you think they will mention it? Apart from having no concept of body awareness, there's a belief in the first-timer that they can keep up with the regular 'gym goer' in the class. Despite having taught several options (beginner, intermediate and advanced) catering for all the levels in the room, it's often the first-timer, pregnant women, the guy with the spinal injury and the person who thinks they can perform the exercise correctly but end up giving a completely new exercise that I've never seen before who attempt the advanced moves! Choose one option people, just one option and stick with it! Instead of watching the instructor, many first-timers tend to watch the people around them and mimic what they see through them. Similar to Chinese whisper, somewhere along the line it's going to go seriously wrong, and before you can say, 'What the fuck are you doing!' there's a cluster of people creating a new trend of some un-orchestrated, never seen before exercise! Who's the teacher? Breathe!

THE CLUELESS!

When arriving for class, there are normally people sitting on the mats waiting for some form of instruction. Trying to be early for classes is ideal but when relying on transport in London, it's not always practical. As I rush into the studio, I may instruct, 'Everybody on all fours, hands under shoulders, knees under hips' as I head for the stereo to put some background music on. As soon as I'm organised, when turning towards the class, there can be around twenty faces staring at me as if I've asked them to count to ten in French. It could be the accent, although my accent has toned down since being in London. It could be the fact that it's been a while since they've been on all fours! In some cases there are those who can't speak English and seem to think they can wing it by looking around the class and copying others! A few clubs rely on me to virtually do the whole class. If I stand up and walk around, there's anguish in the room, a sense of regret for not paying attention to the instructor, a fear of actually having to listen. Most instructors I know teach on average fifteen to twenty-five classes a week. Some unbelievably teach more although that won't last for long. The travelling can be a killer in itself, never mind having the physical strength to demonstrate moves in every class taught and motivate on top of that. Motivating unmotivated people can itself be mentally gruelling. The toughest classes I would say to teach are the beginners'. They require so much guidance in how to stand, sit or lie posturally correct.

In some cases I need to counsel myself not to get upset or worked up, especially if someone can't understand the difference between a pelvic tilt and a pelvic lift. This is after I've demonstrated the moves several times over. For some people, they'll never get it. A lack of wiring from the brain to the rest of the body misreads information, which makes the body move in spasms of uncontrolled movement. A simple action of standing upright can look like one leg is shorter than the other with the chest puffed out and chin squeezed into chest. Standing on both feet – a class in itself!

I do, however, love watching some people perform the bike manoeuvre or in Pilates it's known as the Criss Cross. This exercise is performed lying on the back, fingers behind the head and literally twisting elbow to opposite knee. Some can perform this exercise correctly. Some execute the move in an interesting way. A way that generates new ideas for new moves for myself for future classes. Then there are those who look like a cross between a baby having a tantrum and someone having an epileptic fit. It's an impressive display of a too often exhausting performance, but hey, if they feel they've had a workout, great. There's just no correcting some people. A select few just know what they're doing, the autopilot button is switched on and nothing will convince them otherwise. I often feel exhausted just watching them.

THE WINDED!

Lack of body awareness can pose a problem for the exerciser; however, lack of body control can prove highly intoxicating for the rest of us if an epidemic of farting occurs. Some farts are loud as they reverberate throughout the room shaking the window panes, others are silent but deadly. I can be walking innocently around the room when all of a sudden my eyes cross over in a hypnotic state as I pass through the lingering deadly smell. I'm fortunate to be able to walk away but the poor surrounding bodies on the floor are left paralysed (or is it comatose) to inhale every vapour of the offending gas! When teaching, the tiny princess toots are excusable. I had, on one occasion, a girl who dropped an earth-shattering fart, which I ignored and continued teaching above the stifled laughter. It was a challenge to keep a straight face as the girl trumpeted a second and third time. Whether suffering from IBS or practising to enter the Royal National Orchestra, by this time I wanted to look at her and say, 'Are you quite finished?' The call of human nature can't be helped though and thankfully the breathing during the class was still a practicality! Most classes I've taught, I've managed to avoid chemical warfare. One guy who came to my beginner Pilates class looked as if he lived on protein shakes. I was impressed that all walks of life these days were willing to give Pilates a go to reap the benefits it can offer. On this unfortunate occasion for the rest of us, protein boy unleashed what seemed like a strategic planned attack on the entire room and if the room had no walls, it would've spread to the surrounding buildings too. It was loud, intense and alarming to the point I thought I'd have to plug my nose and breathe through my mouth. Those who have never experienced a protein fart before, be thankful, be very thankful. It can sound like a 747 jumbo jet coming into land and like catching the flu, the eyes water and the nose streams under the changing warming environment caused by the steam inhaled. I never saw him again. Like kids to the playground, farting is a phenomena, which will always lead to an outburst of humiliation or laughter. Words of advice before doing any style of class, predominantly the classes which are heavily focused on the belly area: avoid protein shakes and beans, go to the toilet to decrease any pressure in the abdomen area, lighten the load literally from embarrassing yourself and others and in return it will save the planet from any more toxic gases and the rest of us from burning our noses.

THE PERVERTED STALKER!

From time to time, there can be a rather keen participant who likes to hang around after class to have a general chat. Talking about the moves performed in the class, the benefits of fitness or nutritional advice would be the presumed conversation; however, agenda can vary for everyone. With what seems to be at first an intrigue in the class, swiftly escalates to looking for one-to-one training and with that comes exchange of mobile numbers. Within hours of swapping numbers, the potential new client enthusiastically messages to ask how my day is and if I'd like to meet for drinks before the one-to-one session commences. The simple reply to unwanted potential problems is to use the 'I'm too busy' excuse. It can sometimes easily be identified those who genuinely want to train and those who have the ultimate desire to sleep with their trainer. Questions not involving training are an obvious give away, coupled with glazed expressions on the face.

With profile boards on the gym wall and easy access to mobile numbers, sometimes the anonymous sender can send all sorts of crude messages. In some cases, pictures! It's been known that some PTs have had to change their numbers after receiving anonymous fanatic sexual messages. It's not, however, always the member who initiates the sexual tension. PTs can use their fitness status to their selling point. Wearing clothing that leads little to the imagination. In an environment where image is everything, the PT can utilise the equipment cleverly to open and squeeze parts of their clients for their self-gratification. One PT in a central London gym was notorious for bedding his clients. In fact he probably spent more of his time in bed than he did the gym. More like an escort than a PT, his workouts were definitely varied but evoke a response from the general public about the fickleness of the industry and puts it into disrepute. There are a lot of highly-educated fitness professionals in the industry and it can turn the whole concept of PT into some kind of circus.

THE TEACHER'S PET!

Where there is a classroom situation there are the dynamics between the teacher and the learner. The adult classroom can replicate primary school kids. The non-listeners, the late arrivals, the chatty, the disruptive, the inquisitive, the confrontational to the teacher's pet who, instead of bringing an apple to class for the teacher, sets up the instructor's space whether it be the mat or other forms of equipment. It can be a pleasant change from the negativity that can breed within the gym. Kindness does happen and it can over-shine those who are set on disrupting the dynamics of class life! The teacher's pet will execute every move as instructed by the teacher whether it be swinging the arms over the head to burping in a rhythmic fashion. At the end of the session, the teacher will of course be helped by their pet to put the mats away.

THE CREATURES OF HABIT!

Routine is something we all adopt whether it's waking up at a specific time and having the same breakfast we make for ourselves each morning or going to a particular class at a set time. In the gym, our favourite machines are earmarked and heaven forbid if someone's on them. The studio can have mats or equipment set out in preparation for a class, sometimes thirty minutes before it begins. I can predict before the class commences the set-up of who's going to be where. Shy Sarah, along with the first-timers choose the very back of the room away from the prying eyes of the exhibitionists, fashionistas and the inspiring fitness wannabes who of course are at the front, literally leading the class. SAD-suffering Sally goes near the window in the vain hope of catching any ray of sunshine that will invigorate her through the misery of exercise. The teacher's pet settles near the front but to the side of the class in order to help the teacher with any technical issues like controlling the air conditioning unit, stereo volume or helping with the distribution of equipment. The perverted stalker is located near the back but to the side of the room in order to scope out the whole class for potential dates, mates and for the fact it's near the tissue dispenser to wipe any sweat or drool from their mouth, nose or... Those purely in the room for fitness fill up the middle section. Class complete!

THE PRENTENTIOUS!

In the centre of London, in some of the more prestigious clubs there are the members who seem to think they are above everybody else, so much so they can't believe they're in the same room as themselves. While correcting a lady during a Pilates exercise, she seemed so defensive towards being adjusted that she addressed me with, 'Do you know who I am?'

So, being in my home comforts, the studio, I replied, 'Oh, someone's got amnesia, have you forgotten your name?' Trying to make a joke from it, it created quite a storm in the class as you can imagine. Fellow participants displayed stifled laughs and faces of congratulations as if to say, you put her in her place. I moved away from her and left her to her own devices and continued the class. She stayed for the rest of the class and left without further embarrassment to herself. Job done I think! I never did find out who she was though! Within the same club, there are the ladies who still dress for aerobics as if it's the eighties, and there are some members who treat the class as some drop-in centre, walking in and out as they please, not following the routine and are basically in a land where only Teletubbies come from – la la land! The class paid well, but for the sake of my sanity and to prevent me from being on a murder charge, I had to give it up! Sanity restored!

THE JANUARY CROWD!

After Christmas and New Year have passed, the New Year's resolutions kick in. The desire for a fresh start, new body and new look is first and foremost on many people's agendas, and normally gym memberships sell like hot cakes on a cold day. The regular gym goer and I all know that the 'January crowd' have a shelf life of about two to three months (sometimes less) before the resolutions of going to the gym (and in some cases not going) have been achieved regardless of whether the results have been as successful! Sometimes it's the psychological mindset of having joined the gym that makes people feel better regardless of whether they visit it for a workout or a drink of coffee. An ambiguous statement of 'I've been to the gym' most of the time doesn't always mean had a workout. Most January memberships are cancelled until the following year, and gym life returns to normality yet again. The January crowd are a combination of the first-timer, the clueless and those who lose control of either their bodily functions or how they're able to functionally move! It's great to see people for the first time giving the gym a go with the slight potential of becoming a regular. It is highly frustrating, however, to see the repeat offenders who systematically join the gym around the end of January to then cancel a few weeks later to only rejoin again the following January! What a waste of money for a start – why not just buy a new computer game or something to keep the fingers active at least. It's always pleasing to see an increase in gym usage in January but with it arrives more chaos! Friends who join together mimic those being trained by their PT not fully understanding that the training session their mimicking is personalised to that individual who's receiving the personal training session. Thin-legged Tina may be working on a programme designed by her personal trainer to beef up her legs unbeknown to wide-legged Wendy who is trying to slim them down.

The best place to spectate the January crowd is in the studio, and in particular a Body Pump class. Pump, a Les Mills pre-choreographed programme normally lasts for forty-five minutes to an hour. Most are unaware that the class is predominantly endurance-based training which means one round of squats can last for up to five or six minutes depending on the track. The January group 'in the form of male' tend to observe the weight about to be lifted by the instructor (which is female in this case). Whatever the female instructor is lifting for squats for example, it's guaranteed that the male participant will lift at least that, plus a little extra as after all, he's a man! What tends to follow, and I always recommend if you're a regular gym goer, is to go near the back to get front row seats, at the distress and disorientation caused to the guy who struggles after one minute into the track. A squat can turn into a 'Michael Jackson'-style dance routine whereby every squat elevates the heels off the floor with a verbal 'Shamong' at the top. After three minutes into the track, bearing in mind there are two minutes left to play, the male participant now is displaying facial signs of regret, fear, anguish, trauma and in some cases looks like a stab victim experiencing cardiac arrest! 'How can a girl lift more than me?' is the question that is obviously running through their minds! The true meaning of training is flashing above them with the message to everyone else to start light and build yourself up from there. Out of all the people in the gym or studio, males have to be the worst for not listening or simply believing that they know best! An attitude of, 'if it's not big and heavy it's not worth lifting' is the general agreement between the ill-trained exercisers. Guys eagerly train their chest and arms to the detriment of their lower body and then end up looking like they have the legs of a seven-year-old. This unfortunately isn't just the trait of the male 'January crowd' but the regular gym goer too. For the 'January crowd' who come to the gym but have no idea what they're doing, they would seriously benefit from personal training. Most people abandon the gym through lack of results, normally having achieved little weight loss. A trip to the gym gives reasoning in some minds that the cheeseburger afterwards is perfectly OK; after all they've worked hard for it! Women avoid weight-lifting in fear of bulking up and so miss their full potential to increase their metabolism which will burn extra calories and tone them up at the same time. When March comes around and the monotony of exercise and lack of results combined are highlighted to the January exerciser via the mirror, it's time to cancel the gym membership. Well, at least until next January!

CHAPTER FIVE

WHEN THINGS GO WRONG!

When teaching a class, so many things can go wrong: the stereo, the head microphone, the music, the air conditioning, the bookings (or lack of), the equipment and the participants. Whether inside a classroom situation or facing a one-to-one client, you're looked upon to 'fix the problem!' with the usual method of a sticking plaster! In one west end club I taught at there was a class happening in the studio. It was a busy class in full swing when all of a sudden someone collapsed (presumably through heat exhaustion). The instructor managed to keep the class going, removed the client outside the studio and literally left them in order to get back to the class! Talk about the show must go on! Nothing came of it as embarrassment always leads the client to creep quietly away into the changing room.

Situations in the classroom are always inevitable especially when people and equipment are involved. I taught a yoga class one evening, quite late at night, and I had one too many bottles of water during the day. Why is it yoga or Pilates classes have to be at eight or nine in the evening? Some people want to relax after work. Anyway, I came to the usual finale of the class, the relaxation. During the relaxation, music was playing, and I softly spoke into the microphone and by this time my bladder was about to explode. I looked around the room of around thirty people thinking if I relax, there's going to be a flood. Contemplating, can I wait! I stood up, made my way towards the door and left the room. As I rushed through the gym, I still had the head microphone around my head, clasping my hands around my mouth to divert any background noise. I tried speaking calmly into the microphone, 'Take a slow conscious breath through your nose… ' People in the gym were looking at me with the suggestive thought of, there's a mad yoga teacher running around the gym telling everyone to breathe. I didn't care, my bladder was controlling my mind as I headed towards the disabled toilet. Before I could relax, I had to make sure the microphone was off otherwise they would've heard the cries of, 'Oh, my God, thank God for that, what a relief!' I crept my way back into the studio, sat down and finished off the relaxation. When the class was leaving, I asked a regular attendee and mate of mine, Eli, if she noticed me leave during the relaxation and she said she was oblivious to it all. Result! I was thinking how professional can I be for the fact nobody noticed me leaving. As with most momentous occasions it was a short-lived experience. My mate, David, had great pleasure informing me that during the session whilst demonstrating a wide-leg stretch against the mirror, my trousers left little to the imagination. The class may have been oblivious to my 'bladder crisis,' however, during the session when I had everybody gathered around me, legs propped against the mirror to do a wide-leg stretch, everyone's attention was drawn to the essence of the move. Unknown to me, my trousers around the crotch area fitted rather well, and let's just say, being a male yoga instructor doing a wide-leg stretch with everything on show was a performance in itself. Perhaps a reason for constantly busy class numbers! Note to self – must choose better attire next time and definitely not wear white trousers with black underwear! Dumb and young, I know, but it's a learning curve or perhaps a new fashion statement.

Along with wardrobe malfunctions and like the machines in the gym, the stereo would often not work before class, crap out during class or be stolen after class. With most group fitness classes, music is the key ingredient to a great class, and so as a temporary measure, when the stereo was not operational and until a new stereo from Thailand or some other faraway land arrived months later, a small portable stereo was often the substitute. The small portable stereo was big enough for a small kitchen and had a tinny ring to it with no bass when the volume was turned up. Every movement was recorded via the CD player by it either jumping forwards or backwards one beat. It wasn't very professional, highly irritating and often resulted in me looking up to the clock every five minutes wishing the class to end soon. It's a kind of relief to give up those classes, which rely heavily on music and the stress that comes with it.

TESTING TESTING...

The microphone is a rare sight in many studios as it's often stolen, broken or cracks during every body movement. Teaching classes that play loud music requires the use of a head microphone to save the instructor's voice; however, with many clubs scrimping over purchasing new equipment, the instructor has to blast their vocals throughout a forty-five minute to one hour session. Try doing that over the space of about fifteen to twenty classes per week, and the throat is pretty much ravaged. Some instructors have had to have nodules removed from their throat as a result of straining their voice. No head microphone is sometimes better than having one as when it's faulty, it can sound like the instructor is trying to perform some kind of rap with every second or third word missed out. I'm fortunate to teach Pilates and yoga, as it does not require loud house music reverberating out and therefore the use of a head microphone. Saying that, the members who arrive late for a busy class, who are then forced to squeeze in the back next to the speaker and normally have a hearing problem, are the ones who complain for the fact they can't hear you. They want you to use a head microphone regardless and prance around like Madonna on valium instead of arriving early or moving to a more appropriate location for them to see and hear you!

The most challenging classes vocally are definitely after a visit to the dentist! If a filling has been undergone which of course requires numbing of the gum, there is a guaranteed challenge to speak your own language never mind getting non-native speakers the chance to understand you! 'Good mohning, any inchuees oh pwehnasees' (translated; Good morning, any injuries or pregnancies). Being freelance, time off means no funds, so sometimes teaching under all conditions is necessary even if it does sound like a slurring of words is the presumed result of one too many of the alcoholic variety! Instructors are human, and not every instructor is robotically militant in eating bananas and drinking fruit juice all day! There are times whereby the instructor teaches whilst under the influence. It can be a great hangover cure sweating in a class, whether it's down to fear of being recognised for drinking or just consuming too much the night before and it's simply seeping through the skin.

If it's not the microphone or the voice that's the issue, it's the music. Teaching a class of thirty or so people, you're never going to get the music to everyone's taste, but still there are those who think your iPod should contain every single song ever composed. Some members even advise on what should be played in the next class if the music isn't to their liking. In pre-choreographed classes, some members seem to think instructors love to learn routines all day every day without realising that it takes time to rehearse what is about to be done in the classroom! A new song requires time spent on learning – it's fine, social lives aren't really important anyway!

COOL IT!

The air conditioning, oh, where to begin with this one. Before, during or after a class, it's either too hot or too cold. Normally I don't even get the chance to change the temperature, as some members will take charge of that aspect for me. Half the room want the heat to avoid getting cold, the other half want it cooler so they don't overheat. A small select few, paranoid about sweating during exercising, want it to be neither hot nor cold but would prefer either the fans on to keep the room cool or want the fire door left open (using a fire extinguisher) to circulate the air in the studio. Leave the fire door open, and the manager then complains for jeopardising health and safety and potentially ruining his health and safety record (and potential bonus). Have the air conditioning on in the first place and the model wannabes fear a change in their skin condition. Heaven forbid if cracks appear! The solution is best left up for everyone to fight it out; I'm not getting involved!

Perhaps mini fans per mat placed above like some kind of air conditioning unit in a plane – control at your own mercy!

APPROACH WITH CAUTION!

Participants bring to class an array of drama and dilemmas. I always ask the 'any injuries, pregnancies' question and tend to walk around the room hunting down replies, as people generally tend to shy away from throwing their hand in the air. Saying that, if someone does wave me over, everyone turns to look at them as if some kind of tourist attraction, but without the cameras. Intense glares signify the question on everyone's mind, 'what's wrong with them?' A woman once signalled me over. I crouched down, and as I repeated the question of injuries / pregnancies she was in the process of removing one of her legs. Trying not to collect too many flies with my jaw dropped open, I thought 'interesting situation'. Pilates predominantly requires the use of both legs and arms for the dynamics of working the core. I asked her if she could leave her artificial leg on but she found it got rather clammy during exercise. So we compromised, and she removed her leg during exercises involving upper body and fixed it back on during lower body exercises. It's something you don't learn on a course – how to deal with someone legless, literally speaking. It definitely felt different having to tell a member, 'You'll need your leg for this next one!'

Often during a Pilates class, I'll walk around and correct people to avoid them jeopardising their back, knees or some other part of their body. Unfortunately not everybody feels they need correcting, after all, they have been doing it for years. They've read the 'how to manual' and know what they're doing! There are even those members who like to tell me how it should be done. With a sarcastic tone (as that's the only way to get through to some people), I'll explain what I'm trying to achieve in a particular exercise whether it be stabilisation or mobility. This is where the individual might be familiar with the exercise but not understand the reason behind modifying the move within the exercise, and they're forgetting it's not all about them, there's more than one person in the room. There are those who believe they are advanced, but to look at, and then tell them that they need to stream it back to basics can sometimes feel like chewing on meat that's hard to swallow. A look of 'how dare you say I'm shit, I've been doing this for ages' is written over their face. Years of doing Pilates doesn't mean it's done correctly. The term autopilot comes to mind for many who work an exercise and switch off while they're doing the move. Thinking about what they're having for dinner, the conversation from the previous day to whether they've locked the front door when they left the house runs through the minds of the mentally befuddled! I know this too well as the befuddlement in my mind in my earlier days switched my ears off from listening to the teacher. Focus! Focus on mind with body!

One of the clubs I taught in had a full class of about twenty people, and I was doing my usual rounds of walking the room. I saw one girl doing it wrong, and she hadn't stated it was her first time, so you can only presume they have some understanding of Pilates. Well, she was compromising her body so much so that I placed my hand on her knee to avoid her rocking her hips and jeopardising her back. She replied with a direct venomous tone to her voice, 'Can you get your hands off me please!' Unknown to me she was a Muslim, and with my naivety I didn't realise I'd done anything wrong. It's a quick learning curve.

It did get my back up though, and I replied quickly, 'Is this your first time?'

She answered sheepishly, 'Yes!' I told her if she had mentioned that at the beginning, I could've gone through some key things with her, perhaps some boundaries.

I snarled at her, 'Either alter what you're doing or don't blame me if you can't walk for the rest of the week!' The problem is I see the advert where there's a blame, there's a claim, and I know from first-hand experience that if people injure themselves and deem you responsible, they will have your balls on the chopping board, no hesitation.

It can be tricky and in the fitness arena quite controversial whether a hands-on approach is the right or wrong way. Sometimes it's necessary to lightly tap a knee from collapsing out especially where a move might jeopardise the back. As I found out the awkward way, it helps to be a good judge of who is fine with being corrected and who is not. I guess for those that fear being adjusted should be prodded with a stick or zapped by taser as a measure for reinforced training!

It reminds me of my job back in Dundee (the feeling of 'get away from me') when I was training two women in the studio. I had them both doing walking lunges and one of the ladies felt ill. Straightaway, I stopped the exercise, told her to lie down, got water for her and as soon as she stopped, she felt a little better. I told them that we weren't going to continue the session and that we could do more next time around. Delving into an understanding of why she felt how she did, I discovered that she had no breakfast that morning! This is typical of many exercisers trying to lose weight. Avoid eating and trying to exercise to maximise their weight loss. Unfortunately if there's no petrol in the car, it isn't going to work. They went to get changed, and when they appeared from the changing room, I asked how she was feeling. All good and feeling ready to book in for another session, I advised them both to eat something before they came the next time.

The next day I came into work only to be called in to the manager's office. I innocently walked in and sat down, and the manager at the time, Kaz, started questioning me about the training I did with the two ladies in the studio. Bewildered to be pulled aside for my actions, I explained what I did, what happened, what I did as a result of her not feeling well and advising them both on eating before a session. Kaz had been given the story that I trained them militarily in a boot-camp style resulting in one of the ladies collapsing. She of course knew my background was yoga and Pilates and my way of training was anything but a 'Hitler-style' boot camp. She said to me if the complaint was directed to another PT who was renowned for pushing, pushing, pushing then the story might resonate well with what she had been told by the ladies. Kaz had mentioned both the women wanted to cancel their membership. At that point I felt absolutely gutted, thinking, you try to help people to improve their general health and wellbeing, and they repay you with a punch to the guts. So these ladies used me as a reason to cancel their membership because to pull out of the year contract that they had signed up for, they had to have a valid excuse. The manager, Kaz, refused their reason and thankfully backed me up. I later heard that they tried to terminate their contracts as they were struggling to keep up with payments. I was fuming for the fact I was used as a scapegoat and felt betrayed for helping someone improve their wellness and in the process experienced defamation of my professional character.

I see every experience I encounter, whether good or bad, as a development to my personal being, professional conduct and a great way to harden up the jaw by clenching the teeth with frustration. I had another confrontation in a different gym with a lady who I saw in passing as I walked to the studio. She came to my class a few times, but then I hadn't seen her for some time. She must've had a January season ticket! I stopped and spoke to her asking how she was and if she was planning to come back to the class. She had a lot of problems with her lower back and told me that the doctor had advised her that Pilates was making her back worse. It was the tone and conviction in her voice when describing how her doctor said she was getting worse as if it was my fault. As an instructor, you reflect on yourself questioning if you're in the correct job, if you need to retrain, and it was then that I started to devalue myself. I felt the gun pressed against my forehead as if to say, 'What have you done to me you bastard?'

I logically started to compute in my brain the questions to fire back at her. 'So how often do you do Pilates then?'

She replied, 'I come to your class!'

Thinking to myself, OK, I've established that much, 'How many other times do you exercise or do Pilates?' The answer I received put all logic back in my mind.

'Just your class, once a week!' It wasn't doing Pilates that was making her back worse! It was the lack of attending Pilates that was causing her problem. I explained that in order to help herself she needed to invest a little more time in the gym and by doing once a week was possibly doing more damage than good. I stated strongly to her that a minimum of three if not four times a week would help keep the back mobile and strengthen up her core.

I wanted to grab and shake her, screaming, 'Own your body, don't blame others for your lack of doing!' Also I strongly advised her if she needed an opinion on her back, to seek a physiotherapist or chiropractor, not a doctor. Taking painkillers would just mask the problem and make matters worse. I headed for the studio with my head held high. I thought to myself, that's another piece of useful advice handed out to somebody who either takes it and acknowledges it or just continues with what they think is right for them.

CHAPTER SIX

LOOK AT ME!

Tears, tantrums and tiaras don't always flourish from the participants. Instructors, PTs and other professionals in the business can carry their ego right on their sweatband. Many fitness conventions I've attended can be full of information, fun, new clothes, new ideas, new fitness concepts, the look / the style, and sometimes it can all just be overwhelmingly pretentious. Those specialised in nutrition obsess, not just at these events but on a daily basis, with how much protein they're eating, have they had enough selenium and zinc in their diet, have they had too many carbs, are they drinking enough water and in the process all normally end up ill and stressed with the burden they place on themselves to be healthy. You are what you eat, or perhaps you are how you eat – paranoid, controlled and badly in need of an anal probe to detect any changes in bodily functions and to inject some excitement into their lives. Heaven forbid if a discovery of too many carbs are in the system. Where's the treadmill? It's definitely a case of OCD! Must go to gym! Must have protein after gym! Must make sure to drink plenty of water to keep hydrated before, during and after! Must make sure to have a rest day! Must make sure to work legs on Friday otherwise will end up like an oil rig – large upper body on stilts! Must make sure to get a life and not get on everyone's tits!

I love my coffee, and at one of these big showy conventions, I once said to the group I was associating with that I was going to grab a coffee. I offered to get one for anybody else in the group and their response was like I'd just said I was going to the toilet to do a line of cocaine. How could I fill my system with such chemicals! I guess I should learn from past experience that coffee before doing exercise is perhaps a no-no. Often when I feel exhausted before teaching a class, I devour a double shot skinny latte, which gives me the jitters and a case of verbal diarrhoea but on the same note gives me the energy to deliver a group fitness class, which in some clubs coffee can be a lifesaver. Who needs drugs when you can get high on caffeine! In my reckless younger years, my classes were a detox session from the previous night! Sometimes lack of sleep, if getting any sleep at all, would force me to resort to coffee overdose and an intense concentration in class as a way of not exposing my social life! Beads of sweat in the form of alcohol droplets would trickle down my face to a studio filled with conscientious health and fitness exercisers. Taking part in a fitness class is definitely a hangover cure especially when teaching in front of an enthusiastic bunch of people! It's also a hangover cure for when teaching in front of misery and despair! Looks and comments of 'I didn't know you drink!'

Imaginary retorts of 'I drink because of you, you miserable fuckers!'

The changing rooms at these conventions (and in most gyms) are a place, not for changing but for transforming. Transforming the hair on the legs, shaved to smooth, smearing the fake tan over the body for a healthier bronzed complexion instead of pasty white, a chance to pose in the mirror to investigate any potential fat forming just under the six-pack and to formulate ways to transform it into firm. This is just a normal day in the men's changing room. The male presenters, performing the new classes in front of the multitude of enthusiastic fitness followers, exhibit their smooth chest, arms and legs which blind many of their fellow professionals if the light hits their legs at a particular angle. The legs with what looks like polished shins, military standard, reflect light like a mirror, direct and blinding. Hours of preening and pruning give the celebrity instructor an edge and a reason to be smug on stage as they are the beacon of hope to other wannabes who are then eager to buy the latest DVD and music so they too can mimic their idol. It takes a while to finally identify that the celebrity instructors are not there for themselves. The crowd of followers don't care either way as they struggle to work to the same capacity as their idols regardless of technique. During the show extravaganza a complexion of admiration, stress and anxiety is displayed on the participating faces. Admiration for the hero or heroine standing in front of them but stress and anxiety with a fear that the branded souvenirs on offer to purchase will soon disappear if they don't get in there quickly. Glares from the participants are felt throughout the room as eyes scout the competition, checking on the technique of others and judging the general attire and body image. Thoughts of what is she wearing? Wow, she has a huge ass and what on earth is that move called – a press-up or a let-down! I think the guys are definitely more flamboyant in contrast to the girls for showing off their theatrical performance whilst on stage. Perhaps a missed opportunity to appear in a West End musical!

With every fitness exhibition there follows the fashion industry, from catwalk to combat. The clothes are part of the overall product trying to be sold. Whether the clothing coincides with the physical movement is a contentious issue. Imagine Britney Spears in her red cat suit trying to perform a squat. It's not practical but it's good to look at! The products galore cannot be bought at local retailers and so the prices are hugely inflated for the poor fitness .professional. The desire to replicate their idol is so great, however, that their eyes enlarge to that of an owl when comprehending what to purchase. When I'm in this atmosphere, I envisage many Madonnas impersonating her during her 'Like A Virgin' days – bangles, beads, the hair with clothes ripped and hanging off the shoulder with an attitude of 'I'm too cool for school, fuck you'-kind of look! Sad, but true! Individuality coupled with creativity is morphed into one with the ultimate goal to replicate all those around them!

There was a girl who taught a class at the same time as I taught mine but in the opposite studio. Outside the studio doors whilst waiting for the previous classes to empty, her expression towards everyone was fierce although at first I thought she had constipation pains. She played this awesome ninja role with her camouflage trousers and tight tank top. It became more obvious what class she was doing when she started to wrap her hands with Les Mills branded wraps. For those not familiar with the purpose of wraps, they are used by boxers to prevent injuries and provide wrist support while executing punches to solid objects like a bag or a person. Apparently this woman seemed to think the strength of her punch into open space might damage her hand or wrist during her Body Combat class. Well, if that's what was worn in the DVD, why question it?

DON'T THINK, WATCH!

Fitness has definitely changed over the years since I started within the industry. The years of freestyling and creativity has dramatically shrunk to the detriment of some of the best instructors in the business. Pre-choreographed classes are the 'in thing' at the moment, and I can't completely knock it as I once followed that route and learned many things from doing it. At the end of the day if any type of class can get people out of the cake shop and off their seats to become more mobile and stronger then all praise to them. However, for those fitness professionals who only mimic pre-set routines, they lose a little part of the grey matter in their brains. Copying an original format will always leave them in second place! Think of it like Britney Spears covering a Beyonce track. A hopeful attempt but like a recipe with missing ingredients. There's a lack of understanding in why a certain pattern of movement is how it is; alternatives are there any and if so will it be shown on the DVD or in the notes as my grey matter stopped working years ago and I struggle to think for myself! Is this DVD fitness culture making the modern instructor intellectually challenged? Is doing the same routine for a period of time bringing monotony from the gym into the studio? Can real self-satisfaction be possible for replicating someone else's work? When a new routine is released, you just have to stare at the instructor to see them thinking of the next move or is it the contemplation in their mind that after week two they will know the words to every song played inside out better than the artist singing the song! With some classes there are participants all over the place during the routine but the instructor is too focused on perfecting the formula of movement preset for them to be concerned if anybody is stepping out of line! After weeks of teaching the same routine, mistakes occur with some instructors as they themselves switch off and move to autopilot! Why not learn a new routine? Well, this takes time for those who have more than three programmes to teach, and plus it takes time to select the correctly branded attire to use for the class! I guess the DVD and clothing manufacturers are happy with the potential sales increase however!

You only have to attend these so called workshops to identify the rows of qualified instructors interpreting what they perceive from the ones illustrating the routine as the right way. To look into the studio and watch the performance done by all these qualified individuals is a frightening spectacle knowing that some, if not all of these individuals, will be released into the wilderness to reproduce how they think it should be done to their own followers. The synchronicity of movement against music can look like a cross between waves in the sea and a Mexican wave. Does no one have timing to music! Are they listening to their own music ringing in their heads! Sometimes looking good is achieved by lifting loads of weights, but when the form starts to go, isn't it time to shed the weight and perhaps get a better range of movement instead of a quivering squat! I'm thinking this maybe wasn't mentioned in the DVD or the notes. It'll be told in the next round of workshops. PHEW! Just in time before anyone really does some damage to their back! I've taken part in a few pump classes and regardless of how good the instructor is there are those individual members who would be better suited to one-to-one training instead of group training or perhaps a role as a majorette. Some people just need more time to get it! Whatever it is they're trying to get! Those pump instructors who teach ten or more pump classes a week display great signs of tolerance through hearing the same music time and time again. The excess of doing so many pump classes takes its toll on not just the instructor but also the members' lower back. Repetitions over a period of five minutes per track with varying technique place strain on backs, knees, elbows, neck and ass muscles as it's impossible to breathe through the mouth with gritted teeth and clenched facial muscles. As soon as they stop, their pain subsides.

Most of the general public, who sit behind desks for long periods during the day, accentuate their rounded postures as they slump at their computer screens. Some attend a pump class to hold a straight bar for the duration of around five minutes to work the upper arms. The bar forces them to turn their palms uppermost for the arm track. Some of these attendees are first timers. They've never lifted a weight heavier than their laptop and are now standing in class to work to an endurance level with palms, shoulders and other parts of their bodies forced into positions which are unnatural to them!

Body Pump is a whole body workout but for some it can look like an out of body experience. Track 1; The Warm-Up. An important part to the workout. It prepares the body for what's about to come; however, some see it as a chance to give them extra time to set up their equipment, chat to their mates, fix their hair or to turn up for the beginning of the actual workout (track 2). Normally the first-timer, pregnant and the injured fall into this category of latecomers, especially after the instructor has explained alternatives for those with special conditions and what to expect from the class. The clueless load up the bar as if competing for some bodybuilding championship competition even though advised by the instructor what weight they should roughly lift. A few minutes into the track signs of struggle are emphasised through posture and facial expressions. False smiles of confidence and strength are displayed under eyes of pain and anguish.

Track 2; Squats. A phenomena not understood by many and that's including some instructors. A squat is something that many guys tend to avoid and, if attempted at all, can resemble ducking under a door – a small bob down and up. A select few manage to come up on to their tiptoes (perhaps with the aim to strengthen ligaments in their toes) and others can be seen rounding their backs as if auditioning for 'the Hunchback of Notre-Dame'. Depending on the speed of the music will depend on the execution to the squat. I always found the faster squatting movements kicked right into my lower back no matter how much I changed my foot positioning. The hovering squats are by far the most laughable especially when looking around the room and observing what seems to be a mass of chronic constipation sufferers. Wrongful cues from the instructor of weight on the heels can cause untold pain to many a follower. Imagine a five-foot person in comparison to a six-foot-five person – whose ass will stick out the furthest when shifting their weight on the heels whilst performing a squat? How will this feel for the back of the tall person? One rule for everyone, I think not!

Track 3; Chest. The advantage of working chest whilst lying on your back is that it can be bounced off the chest at a speed similar to a crash test dummy into a crash barrier. Those with breast implants create extra bounce with momentum. Like the squat, range of movement can be the challenge here. Holding the bar above the head without bending the arms much is a common sight as if trying to hold up a falling roof. Arching the back off the bench is also common and really should be left for the yoga classes; however, it could be an additional stretch for the limited or lack of stretching in the final (stretch) track. It may also be a new way to create storage space in some of the cramped studios whereby your head literally rests on someone else's groin.

Track 4; Back. When doing overhead presses, lifting the bar from waist to shoulder height can look like attempting to throw a small child over the head. The 'Hunchback of Notre-Dame' returns for the rowing action, which can also look like a sweaty pervert rubbing their hands up and down their thighs in quick succession.

Track 5; Triceps (back of arms). Similar to the chest, the bar can bounce off the body in this track. When taking the bar to the forehead the elbows can often widen to the size of football goal posts. If dipping off the side of the bench, too often the shoulders get a good workout as a result of fear in dropping the butt too low in case it gets burnt by an imaginary lit match held underneath. The legs also get a good workout, probably more so here than in the squat or lunge track!

Track 6; Biceps (front of arms). The classic arm curl tends to work everything but the bicep. Swinging is normally the first action to occur to gain momentum to lift the weight up. The second is arching the back similar to the chest track but from a standing position. It's also the second rendition of the yoga back bend. The chest and the biceps coincide here as a favourite for the male species, not just in a pump class but also outside in the gym. There's a necessity to load up the weight particularly in this track

Track 7; Lunges. Another leg track and executed with a unique style similar to the squats. Imagine a sandpit in front of you and without jumping, you have to step over it. Welcome to the lunge track. If not that extreme it's the opposite, stepping over a pencil perhaps with the upper body bowing forwards and knee shooting beyond the front foot. Somehow the back leg seems to spasm and lock in a straight position regardless of what the front leg does!

Track 8; Shoulders. A weak part of the body for many people and normally the legs get a good workout here. Probably more so here than in the squat and the lunges. The upper back tends to lean so far back to press the bar to the ceiling that it resembles a Keanu Reeves 'Matrix' style back bend!

Track 9; Core (belly). Similar to biceps, everything but the core can get worked here. If the neck had a six-pack then there would be a lot of ripped necks out there.

Track 10; Stretching. The finale to the class, the icing on the cake and at times can feel like thin icing! The stretching element often feels rushed and is a clear indication to the participant that it's time to tidy away the equipment. A class of twenty participants can end up being ten actually doing the stretches. Most people tend to have tight muscles; however, it looks cringeworthy when seeing the instructor, the leader of the pack, struggling to reach for their toes. At least style it out if it's your weakness instead of slouching and thrusting head forward with a long neck in a type of 'E.T. sequel 2' film.

Les Mills has had a major influence on the fitness industry and everyone who attends a gym or fitness centre will have come across the various Les Mills brands. Body Combat, Body Pump and Body Balance to name a few have well structured programmes with identifiable criteria within each discipline. They attract the masses, and it's been fantastic to get 'asses into classes'. The prerequisites are to have a gym or aerobics certification. The training takes around three days and then a time limit is given to submit a recording of the whole class being performed in front of a group of participants. A judgement is made on the whole performance and a pass or 'try again' option is delivered back to the trainee.

I used to teach the Body Balance programme. A mixture of tai chi, yoga and Pilates choreographed to what I think is great inspiring music. The unusual concept that I never quite grasped was the presenters or individual instructors who teach this (individual instructors who are not qualified in yoga, Pilates or tai chi) state that its moves inspired from these disciplines, but it's not yoga, tai chi or Pilates! The baffling thing is that when performing the moves, the names are exactly the same as the moves used in the disciplines – down dog, warrior one, warrior two, tree pose are a few of the recognised moves used within the programme. I guess it's a safeguard to say, 'Hey, I'm not a yoga instructor, I'm not a Pilates instructor, I'm a group exercise instructor!' At the end of the day it has stretching in it, core work in it regardless of whether you are Pilates / yoga qualified. My point is that executing stretches and core work requires background knowledge to understand what part of the body needs to be adjusted or fixed in order to feel a move in a more productive way. Picture sitting on the floor with the legs stretched out in front with the aim to touch the toes, i.e., my first session in yoga. Lack of understanding will result in rounding the back to reach for the toes; the pelvis tilts back to further exacerbate the roundedness within the spine. A more productive way, especially for most of the general public, would be to sit on a folded towel to allow the alignment of the pelvis and to help the tipping from the hip not rounding from the spine. Bent legs will help the over stretching of the back of the legs as most people are tight in this area! Add music and a time factor to perform this move along with grabbing a towel and correcting, verbally, the thirty people in the room along with the options for the pregnant girl, the guy with the herniated disc and the group of beginners hiding in the back – oops, next move! 'You'll get it next week stick with it!' A class for everyone, I think not! You can explain and go through options at the start of the class in the vain hope that people will remember but more often than not when teaching a class to music people get lost in the moment. One pregnant woman becomes a class of pregnant people. At the front you see a mob of people, one copying another, whereby something goes wrong somewhere along the line. 'NO, this is the pregnancy option; this is the move you guys need to do. NO, this move is not for you; remember I told you the pregnancy option was this! Forget it, next move! Oh, and remember to breathe!' Body Balance along with other Les Mills programmes are great only if they have the correct ingredient – a knowledgeable instructor of that field and one who can adapt the program to fit to their audience! When I did Body Balance, I had no tai chi training behind me. I flowed through the routine, clueless of the concept behind the moves but following the pretty music and the feeling of well it must be doing something. If there was a tai chi instructor around, I would've asked them, but then it's not tai chi we're doing so I'm kind of screwed either way. Wing it I guess and remember to smile!

To enhance my instructor ego, my class often asked where else I taught and if they could get my autograph (oh, hold on that's just in my head). They reaffirmed with me a noticeable difference between instructors even though it was the same discipline being taught. Intrigued and needing a further boost to my ego, I would ask what's so different about the teaching styles? A few struggled to conclude the reasons, but others divulged that the explanation of the technicality of the moves and the ability to make subtle movements in order to change the dynamics of the move made the class a class of its own. I'd sometimes alter the choreography to suit the calibre of people I was teaching. An older group would have a tougher time keeping up during the core track for example, and so I'd modify the moves or remove an exercise in order to spend longer on a particular move. Does the 'modern instructor' realise this is possible or are they forgetting that patience is a virtue and it could be mentioned in the next training DVD!

Attending the quarterly workshops for Balance was like watching a second rendition of Pump. The people taking part were all at different stages of the routine. Heads were bobbing up and down like meerkats to confirm the move performed by the lead instructor while listening for the instructions. The competitive within the room were challenging themselves against the 'real' yogis. Everyone trying to be posturally correct but looking posturally strained by trying so hard to look their best. The workshop, supposed to be educational, normally consisted of working through the same routine, which is reproduced on DVD. Just give us the goddamn DVD or at least give some correctional work on positioning during the workshop. At least something to help the non-yoga and non-Pilates people in the room. Some yogis however can be a little too postural as they hyperextend their lower backs as if to flare their feathers like a peacock in mating season. Words of, 'This is my domain, back off and watch me!' etched all over their face. OK, look flexible by not overworking it. We know you can get your leg over your head but at least get some core about you and pull your belly in. It's group fitness not Ashtanga yoga, and besides, a large chunk of the population can't even straighten their legs without untold pain so reel it in! Perhaps they've missed their vocation in performing arts or Cirque du Soleil so there's a desire to perform to the confused public!

So to top it all, the inspiring copycat instructor who attends the modules to qualify, who acquires the DVD and music to learn and play within the class, who attends quarterly workshops to keep their qualification up to date and who normally does more than one programme has to pay for the entire privilege! Now, I'm no accountant but surely on the profit and loss sheet it's going to look something like profit made from classes, losses made from DVD, CD and quarterly workshop attendance! The more amusing side is that instructors who teach this style of class wonder why they're often skint! I'm thinking the next course to study should be maths or business management!

Fitness crazes come and sometimes thankfully go. Zumba a style of dance class has been a huge instalment to the industry and attracts millions of participants. It's turned older women's dress sense into something resembling fifteen year olds on acid. To become qualified as an instructor in the past, there have been no prerequisites. Both dancers and fitness instructors alike may be attracted to enrol on a Zumba course to add an extra string to their bow and an extra pound to their bank. The general public and the addictive Zumba goers can all qualify as an instructor by simply attending a prior workshop to train in the steps used within the programme itself. My mate, Diego, teaches Zumba, and I've taken part in his class. He's a fantastic 'freestyle' instructor with creativity and an abundance of energy on his side. He has an array of other disciplines to his belt making him clued up in body awareness and movement. Unfortunately this is not the case for other Zumba instructors. Anatomy and physiology is not a necessity to train as a Zumba instructor, so the components of the class may be the same for every class one person attends, but the logic, reasoning and thought behind a class routine may differ from a highly experienced and educated instructor to the ones who only do the one or two day course. I guess even a kid can do it using their knowledge of the song 'head, shoulders, knees and toes, knees and toes!' Teaching Pilates during the Zumba era, I've had many of those who declared they hurt their back while participating in this latest craze were either first-time or

131

regular Zumba participants. Was it the 'off the street' instructors that caused it, the well equipped with knowledge and experienced instructor or was it for the fact it's a Latin-style class where hips should be able to have a mind of their own and not everybody has hips like Ricky Martin or Shakira? A clued-up instructor would know of adaptations and progressions to enhance an individual person's workout and be able to use this within a mixed ability group. It's group fitness after all! The not so clued-up – well, let's just say they're trying to get the sixty-year-olds to grind their ass to the floor in some Miley Cyrus twerk competition. Professional dancers who teach Zumba should never be hired in the fitness industry! As a group fitness manager at the time I'd hired a girl who was a professional dancer teaching Zumba. If an audition came up for the potential dance wannabe then she would simply abandon the class at the gym and not even courteously consider the members and myself by letting anyone know. It happened several times before I axed her, having honoured her excuses several times and received enough abusive emails (and quite rightly so) from members.

It's easy to distinguish Zumba instructors from the general public. There's an impulsivity to wear rubber bracelets which at first you'd think it was their devotion to finding a cure for cancer. On the bracelet is the word 'ZUMBA', and even though it's a cheap way of buying jewellery, it can't smell good after a few classes surely. Well, I guess it's more money in the pocket for the guy who invented it and like a dog to its collar, saves one from getting lost! Another obvious feature is the dress sense. Whether looking like heading for a Wham concert or it's the required thing to do, there's a must with all Zumba instructors to wear neon clothing. It doesn't just stop at bright colours but wearing makeup too. How's it possible to not look like a car crash with sweat flying all over the place! If it's not the unique appearance, it's the Tourette's during the class. Shouting out 'Zumba' at several occasions of the lesson makes you wonder if the instructor's reminding themselves or everybody else that they're doing a Zumba class! Is it really necessary? Maybe I should try it throughout my class, 'PILATES!' The music in Zumba can be fun when in the mood but for most of the time it gives me a burning desire to reach for the nachos with extra guacamole. This can be the case especially when I see the instructors move as if they have artificial hips. How do the rest of the class manage or are they thinking nachos too!

THE NEW RECRUITS!

After many years in fitness it's presumed the next phase is to teach or assess the 'new' teachers! I went on my teacher-training and assessing course to learn how to teach other fitness-style courses to potential instructors and to also assess those awaiting release into the industry. Like being at the optician's it was definitely an eye opener to the calibre of people being accepted on the courses and subsequently pumped in the masses into the fitness arena. How do you assess stupidity? Anybody can be accepted onto a fitness course and this is evident when standing faced in front of a classroom full of unmotivated, uninspired, gormless delinquents who look like they've just stepped off the stage from the 'Jeremy Kyle show'! In the age of technology, texting, facebooking and other social media, some people have difficulty in communicating on a face-to-face level, LOL. I taught a fitness instructor course, and there was one twat who stood out. He asked the question 'Is smoking cannabis all right if you still exercise?' How do you respond to that? Was doing the course for him a means of something to do, nothing on the TV and a step up from benefits? Out of a group of twenty individuals, about a quarter of them had the potential to achieve success in a demanding industry. Enrolling on these fitness courses with the desire to become a fitness trainer and then charge £50 plus per hour is far more appealing than applying for a supermarket job whereby you wear some dodgy uniform with a dog collar and get paid around £7 per hour. The amusing thing is a lot of people do not realise the volume of work entailed in completing a fitness instructor course. This is evident in the aerobics course where you'll find some of the girls flapping around in tears as if going through a break up with the boyfriend not quite meeting their expectations. Well, it's the same for aerobics – not quite meeting the expectations and having to learn anatomy and physiology and not just jump around to pretty music! Some people on the course were utterly stressed before actually setting foot through the studio doors. When it came to teaching in front of the rest of the group, people would simply fall apart. Focusing so much on the beats of the music and forgetting the process to teach, coach, instruct, encourage, pre cue and everything else that comes with being a group fitness professional. A few people would simply abandon the course (in a traumatic state I may add) with the realisation that it's not for them.

To have only a fitness instructor or aerobics course on the CV is not enough if you want to be successful in the industry. A huge investment in time, commitment and money is essential to progress within a competitive field. It's annoying to hear of people bored with their office jobs and then deciding the easy way to make good money is to become a PT or group fitness instructor. Not everyone is cut out for the fitness industry, and some people have a very blind view of the difficulties involved within the industry in order to be successful.

As for assessing these courses, it's like assessing someone in accident and emergency! Where do you begin! In an aerobics assessment, as long as the candidate ticks the health and safety boxes they're ready to work in a health club. This is regardless of whether they can string choreography together. To watch these future potential instructors is painful. To think that they could be the next clan of instructors teaching people on how to make their bodies work better is a scary reality. To enter the industry is to simply have the infamous 'passion' for fitness regardless of many factors! Some people have rhythm, others live in denial that they have rhythm and as for the rest, well, it's like watching a male bodybuilder wear high heels; it can all be rather cumbersome. Many of these courses should be more stringent on who they accept to enrol, but of course it's a paying customer. Who can refuse cash and profitability! In order to make the course provider look good, it's essential to get 100% pass rate so that others will take up their courses! Failure for the training provider is not an option so in order to make 'Mr IQ of 50' more impressionable, make him wear a suit to mask the flaws of his two left feet! Get him to resit the exam again and again until a pass result is scraped! Following on from my experiences and observations, I couldn't face being part of the acceptance process. I couldn't pass everybody on a course when I felt they were nowhere near ready for helping others to improve their fitness and wellbeing. I abandoned the idea of becoming a teacher or an assessor. I didn't want to hear of somebody being passed by me injuring somebody else!

CHAPTER SEVEN

NEW MANAGEMENT!

Change is good, or so we are led to believe by the person making the changes. With every new management there comes change, and with change it often entails a serious shafting up the ass with a huge aubergine or a bang to the head through some form. There can be frustration to change when things are working well. In some cases it might be a simple and welcomed change like replacing the empty toilet rolls with ones full of paper, unblocking blocked toilets or water coming out from the water fountain – and this is a big deal in gym life! Especially for the high-protein consumers with their regular toilet visits and fitness-conscientious obsessive compulsive disordered intent on consuming their regular quota of water intake.

Moving machines around and adding more rules and procedures to the already growing Magna Carta of gym politics is an unwritten necessity to the new gym manager. A burning need to put their individual stamp on the club and to satisfy their feeling of 'it was me that transformed this club' flaring their chest as they pound hard on it, Tarzan-style. Some clubs take bookings for classes and then remove this to make it first come first serve. A new manager then starts within the space of two years (which tends to be the trend) and feels compelled to introduce a token system whereby class participants receive a token for a class to guarantee their place. I've never come across any gym that has found a system which actually works. If the procedure is booking for a class then people will naturally book for it; however, they don't always turn up for the class. Prior engagements like a bar crawl are far more appealing! This means classes look busy on paper but are quiet in the studio. It's unfair for other members who'd like to attend a class but don't because the space has already been reserved. It's an unfair black mark against the instructor teaching the class in an arena where low numbers mean, you're shit, you're out, no excuses! With classes requiring tokens for entry, people who collect these at reception don't always hand it over to the instructor. Although the instructor will aim to collect them in at the start of the class (if they can be bothered), there are the sneaky few who creep into class, literally army-crawl style, without giving up their tokens or having no token in the first place. People hold on to their tokens like the ring held by Smeagol in Lord of the Rings, My Precious! Tokens, which are kept of course, can be used for next time and create the problem of classes being over subscribed for future classes. Some clubs use different tokens for different days to avoid individuals reusing the same tokens time and time again, but still members find a way to get around it. Are they sleeping in the studio cupboard along with the mats until the start of their next scheduled class? The other method is first come first serve. As one class finishes and another is about to begin there is a cross between happy hour at the bar and 'Boxing Day sales at the shops'-kind of stampede that can occur for a studio class. Throw in an instructor, male or female, who wears tight hot pants and it becomes a rock concert within a busy train. Strongest elbow wins.

Many group fitness managers like the thought of freelancers managing their own classes by trying to promote their class by whatever means necessary! There was a club I taught at, whereby the instructor would promote the start of his class over the tannoy at reception for the whole gym to hear. 'Abs class in the studio in five minutes, ladies get wet, get ready!' Apart from the Brazilian enticing the women into his wet 'n' wild abs class through his seductive tone and good looks, he also wore the type of outfit which left little to the imagination. Literally you could see the geography of his testicles through his shorts. Wearing tighter hot pants than Kylie Minogue, he managed to pack the class. Although I was dubious whether it was the workout that was actually pulling in the crowds or the fact that the former stripper had a package bigger than what Santa could offer. I guess the physically unfit to the sexually frustrated were challenged in many ways!

No matter how new, ambitious or vocal a new manager can be, a vast majority of gyms are stingily reluctant to hand out the cash when it's greatly needed. Machines that breakdown are removed and replaced with mats or chairs creating space in the gym. I can only conclude the newly formed space are 'thinking areas' or perhaps where some PTs can hunt for unsuspecting prey or lounge around waiting for their next appointment to finally arrive. Space as I've mentioned can be a contentious issue in gyms, but a new trend is evolving whereby machines are being replaced by suspension rope, otherwise known as TRX. PTs who have been using these functional methods for some time are joined by the trend following PTs who want to modernise their training and spice things up for their clients. This is instead of the usual thirty-minute run on the treadmill followed by chest and arm exercises. Balls and bags are lifted into the air and thrown to the floor in some new kind of protest against exercise workout. Why not just have a pillow fight! There's reason for some to do these particular types of exercises; however, for others, it simply looks good.

It's well known that gyms and their studios have equipment that is often broken, well-used or not there at all as it's been stolen via the back door fire escape. Well-used yoga mats when lying face down can be the equivalent to parking your nose next to a dog's ass. A mixture of sweaty feet and gaseous emissions make a lovely cocktail just right for the nose. Some club mats are made of foam and strangely have chunks taken out of them – perhaps a missed breakfast or two has resulted in someone eating them during or just after a class. New mats have been ordered though, or at least that's what we've been conditioned to say to the members to keep them at bay and to save management any further stress!

Young managers, who are wet behind the ears, walk around the gym on the second day of the job planning how they can architecturally change their surroundings! Knocking down walls to create new space and a new vibe is met with a look on the freelancer's face of 'you're not from around here, are you?' I'm not going to hold my breath, as I'm not going to win this bet! Weeks then months pass and the only addition to the gym is paper found in the printer and pen lids without the pens at reception! As the two-year sentence comes to an end for the once-budding, now mentally retired and withdrawn, general manager, it's evident through postural assessment that it's time to move to a new club whereby the luxury of having ink is provided within the printer. If the move is executed correctly and to the right location, it may be coloured ink!

ON THE ROAD AGAIN...

The life of a freelance fitness professional can be gruelling at the best of times when we have to trudge from A to B all over the town. Living in London adds the extra burden of relying on tubes and other methods of public transport that work on a good day. Tourists can slow us down en route to the next class making it feel like we're walking in reverse.

Large groups of tourists stand covering the full expanse of the pavement forcing us to walk on the road, to then be run down by a bus or cyclist. Charity workers on the streets, and in their hordes, target individuals who look as if they have time on their hands or simply capture their look of avoidance. Their warm smile from ear to ear like some Cheshire cat attracts your attention. This is before a hand gesture of acknowledgement towards you forces you to grab your mobile and thrust it to your ear to answer a call that's not even there. 'Sorry, I'm on the phone!' It sounds harsh, but if I stopped and invested my time and money into every charity that I'm approached by, then I would be seeking the help from some charity myself or perhaps become an ambassador for charities. Once I've finally reached my destination, I approach the reception hoping that it's still the same management and staff on the front desk so I don't have to explain myself with regards to who I am (I really need a T-shirt with 'STAFF' emblazoned on it). In some places, I'm close to bringing in my passport to prove, yes, it is I. It's maybe an explanation to why there are chunks taken out of the foam mats! Instructors keep a chunk of mat so on arrival to the club it can be shown as proof that they work there! A kind of fit the jigsaw into the puzzle type security measure! The reception staff, like the gym rules, seem to change more than I do my clothes. Some weeks I'm expected to sign in, other weeks I'm told not to bother; if asking for the studio folder to sign my class numbers in, it's often met with a look of, 'WHAT STUDIO, WHAT

FOLDER, THERE ARE NO PENS' or some other clueless response. There's a general lack of communication from top down resulting in headless chickens flapping about reception. God help the new starters behind reception.

Without fail, in the studio folder there's always a reassuring note from the studio manager;

Dear instructors

I want to thank you all for your hard work and just wanted to say keep it up, we highly appreciate what you do for us (note; here we go again). It's been brought to my attention that people aren't doing this or that! (note; and the list goes on to the point you switch off halfway through the dissertation of writing).

In the years spent teaching you could virtually read ahead of the letters left for the instructor before you even see the words 'ATTENTION INSTRUCTORS!' In a role which requires you to motivate and inspire people, the people within the business manage to attack your enthusiasm with every action you do and every rule stipulated by them. Most of us are in the profession for the love and passion of fitness. The introduction of new rules and new egos, however, create the further burden to somebody who just wants to teach the frigging class. A new rate of pay normally comes into force when new management are introduced. A raise of my middle finger towards the management is more likely than a rise to my hourly rate of pay. Unfortunately many clubs lose great instructors, as they just don't reward them well for servicing their members. I have many friends in the industry who feel isolated and undervalued as a freelancer. Some clubs have this ideology of prestigiousness whereby they expect us to turn up for club meetings when they specify. If we can't make these gatherings, there's uproar of disbelief and a 'telling off' for not being part of the team. When there's a club meeting, the freelancer can be considered part of the team. When there's disrepute between freelancer and member, we're on our own! There's no sense of solidarity.

TIME OUT...

When taking much needed time away from the fitness industry in the form of a vacation, it can feel like filling out a visa application or what I imagine it to be like. Finding a cover instructor can be a laborious task. Are they on the cover list of that particular club, are they qualified, are they reliable and are they free to help out? These are just a sample of thoughts that process through the mind of an instructor before even contacting them. I once got cover for a class I taught at Gym Rules. Their policy is if your cover fails to turn up, you get penalised financially for it. I took a measly five days off from work out of the whole year and spent it in London as I'd spent loads of cash that year on my own personal projects, a website, DVDs and article writing to name a few. I courteously emailed the group fitness manager about the class that I had cover for, the name of the cover, their number and that they were on the cover list so therefore a presumption of them being fully qualified, insured and reliable. It's every instructor's dread to receive a call from any club while having much needed recuperation time to refuel and reload for the next round of physical and motivational teaching. On this occasion, I received a call on a Tuesday at 1.05p.m., the class started at one p.m.. Instantly, I knew Houston had a problem. The manager, sounding dazed and confused, asked me the whereabouts of the cover. I pondered and thought does she know the whereabouts of the prime minister, hardly! I was told there were many pissed-off members, and that she had to deal with it. I thought to myself, you're the goddamn manager, MANAGE and frustratingly replied to her with words to the effect of, 'I followed your protocol as per contract, do you want me to baby sit these professionals you have on your list and prod them with a fork to remind them to move their ass when needed?'

Her response: 'You should call them on the day to remind them!'

By this time, I'm losing the will to live. 'Are you fucking joking, so if I'm in the US you expect me to make an international call to remind them to have their breakfast, burp them, then tell them "off to class now or else!"'

The call ended with a non-conclusive reply of, 'Well, this is a mark against you, two strikes and you're out.' Shocked at the call, I hung up thinking, leave it, she's having a bad day and needs to seriously stop wearing her ovaries on the outside. I wasn't fussed about losing the class as I wasn't short of work. I taught there as I loved teaching the vibrant bunch of people that came to the class. I tried to get a hold of the cover instructor and eventually tracked her down. She'd lost her phone and was profusely apologetic for the mishap. She offered to and called the general manager of the club to explain the situation. End of story, or at least I thought it was. When I received the remittance form from the club listing classes taught and classes paid, there sat the penalty notice. Fuming from frustration, I took a deep yogic breath and calmly withdrew my laptop and started tapping furiously away at the keypad. It felt like poetry in motion typing the words 'thanks for the remittance form, however, stop being a tight ass or I'll axe the class,' or nicer words to that effect. I received an email from the group fitness manager a few days later apologising about the situation and reimbursing me the penalty charge. Although the apology was short lived as the paragraph that followed stated that I should communicate to them in a less aggressive and condescending way. Like a red rag to a bull, and I knew I shouldn't respond to such an email, but I couldn't let it sit, so I replied back. I thought to myself if you're reimbursing me (goodwill gesture, I think not) because you're in the wrong (more likely reason) and for the fact that calling cover instructors on the day was not mentioned within the contract, then it's a good job I fought my ground, otherwise I would have played victim to the penalty. Job done! No more emails!

Finding cover can ignite many issues from all concerned. On one occasion, when I took much needed time off, I'd managed to get somebody to cover my Pilates class. I came back feeling re-energised to hear, as I always do, of stories of who was covering this class or that class. When teaching twenty classes or more there can be many covers for many classes in many clubs. In some instances, the cover doesn't show by either forgetting or losing their mobile. Some members are very particular with the instructor who covers the class. The cover instructors always have a hard time temporarily replacing the permanent instructor to the dislike and sometimes acceptance of the member. I normally always receive feedback in regards to who covered me, and with one class they had told me that my replacement had dissed my style of teaching. I could feel the hairs on my back stand up, my claws sharply grew and I was spitting venom. The cover instructor told the members that she was teaching 'real' Pilates which made me think well, what exactly does she think I'm doing then? I approached her face-to-face and had it out with her but she refuted the allegation. Supposedly the whole class must've misinterpreted what she said in regards to bitching about me! There can be snobbery in the world of Pilates and yoga. Claims that the 'real' Pilates are done in a particular way as learnt on the course. Unfortunately when people do a course, there seems to be an inability to apply concepts of a discipline within exercise in general and other areas in life. I often love when confronted with die-hard Pilates enthusiasts who deplore my concept of Pilates teaching. 'This isn't Pilates? Well, what is Pilates to you?' As long as there's a justifiable excuse for doing things, who can really truly argue. I may not always be right, but I'm never wrong or words to that effect! If at the end of the day your back is feeling better, then there must be something correct with my teaching!

AUDITIONS...

When searching for new places to teach in, most gyms go by recommendation from other clubs, or in some cases the members will soon say if the instructor teaching their class is bollocks or not. In my years of teaching group fitness, I've rarely been to an audition but for those that I have attended it's been an interesting 'X Factor' extravaganza. Before the start of the performance, the mentor often poses the questions: How many years experience and who was the training provider? Each candidate displays about five minutes of instructing in front of fellow participating candidates. Sometimes there can be two people observing or just the one, and it's often the group fitness manager of the club present. In the auditions I've attended, it's been interesting to see the exercises some instructors have chosen to highlight their technical competence. Counting each repetition of an exercise does not demonstrate anything apart from missing your vocation as a primary school maths teacher. For those demonstrating technical competency, it can be shocking to watch their lack of technicality when exhibiting the move in question. Surely you would choose an exercise that can be performed gracefully and accurately by yourself and hide your weaknesses at this precise moment in time. Choose something that the rest of the class can follow with ease so that it doesn't become a dog's dinner with arms and legs all over the place. Some allow their egos to creep in and decide to demonstrate the most challenging of moves purely to show off how supple or strong they are. This can be to their detriment as not everyone (although, all instructors) may be at that level, and then the instructor leading the group often shoots themselves in the foot with the inability to teach the class in how to perform the move itself. It becomes more of a 'look at me' situation instead of proof that they can actually instruct!

The assessor overseeing the audition may have some group fitness background and in some cases may only follow the modern style instructor approach with everything pre-choreographed via DVD! When it comes to freestylers demonstrating their Pilates, yoga and Zumba skills to name a few in front of the 'DVD assessor', how on earth can they be critiqued by someone who can only reiterate what is being produced on disc format? I could skip on one leg, waving my arms in distress convincing the assessor that this is modern Pilates, how would they know any better! If they are convinced by intuitive marketing ploys to buy DVDs frequently, then surely I can convince them that even playing twister is a multitasking way of doing yoga and Pilates combined!

CHAPTER EIGHT

THE GOOD, THE BAD AND THE GODDAMN UGLY!

On my travels as a freelance fitness guru, I've seen a vast amount of interesting things happen within the gym. I'm talking about the contrast between highly skilled, professional PTs to the other wannabe, 'what the hell are they doing'-type PTs! If you regularly go to the gym and observe the dynamics of gym life, you'll know exactly what I'm talking about. The 'dodgy' PTs can sometimes be obvious to spot either physically or mentally and in some cases both! It can all begin even before exercise commences. I was in the changing room one day before a class and noticed a young guy getting changed. He was pale looking, very flabby and looked gormless (he just had that look if you know what I mean). He was getting changed ready for a workout to tone those flabby bits up, and I thought 'good on him'. It was only when I saw him slide over his head a T-shirt with the words 'personal trainer' emblazoned on it that I thought, surely it's a gimmick T-shirt and not the real thing? Nope! Fresh off the press, fresh from PT academy he was ready to get people fit regardless of HIS fitness levels.

Should it really matter if a PT preaches fitness but doesn't do it themselves? Should it not be a matter of practice what you preach? He might've been qualified to the highest level, but surely you need to look the part, it is FITNESS PROFESSIONAL after all! You are what you sell. Some members looked more the part than what he did and his posture was shocking – more like a stroppy, tall teenager, slouching with each stride! Perhaps a part of the course that he'd missed.

On the other end of the spectrum and it's not always the case, but physically speaking the overinflated muscle Marys are all muscle with no connection between muscle and brain. There's either a blockage through protein overload or a lack of understanding with lifting heavy weights without due thought to the mechanics of the body and the individual. I hear and see it regularly; the skinny guy approaches muscular PT guy. Skinny guy has an ambition to be like PT guy or maybe not so pumped, 'Men's Health' front cover model, perhaps. A discussion between the two tends to gear mentally around upping the protein consumption by ingesting buckets of the stuff and lifting heavy weights to 'beef up.' No thought for skinny boy having no body awareness whatsoever and the inability to carry his own body without dislocating his shoulder (some city boys really are designed for office jobs, not heavy manual labour). Session one consists of the infamous bench press, some back work and who cares about legs – they tend to be worked slowly on the treadmill at the start of the workout as part of the warm-up, or can be done in one's own time or just wear baggy pants. During the session, the PT needs to have his phone by his side all the time, literally held in his hand by his side, to receive the deluge of calls he's anticipating through the immense demand he has generated with his physique, knowledge and expertise. Of course this is the case, it wouldn't be right to text his girlfriend messages and frequently update his Facebook status! Besides, where would he find the time whilst frequently looking in the mirror at himself instead of his paying client! OK, maybe he's allowed to have a sneaky look at his physique so he can work out his next programme for himself, trim that tiny, little bit of body fat forming just above the waistline. The glare in the mirror might constitute the same glare the girl PT does at the television when training her client. It's a prolonged stare, and judge me if I'm wrong, but there's an intensity to it which demonstrates that these PTs are thinking of the best exercises for their paying client and formulating the best nutrition plan for them surely. If it's not television programmes or iPhones these PTs are concerned with, it's the talent parading the gym floor. Scantily-clad exhibitionists, who come to the gym to show their seductive clothing and toned frames (and occasionally work out), catch the eyes of those pervy PTs, who, for some, make it their daily task to scout for 'eye candy' (individuals who are pleasing to the eye). In some gyms, which can be heavily dominated by male PTs, there can be a playground style atmosphere, fun for some and intimidating for others. Some male PTs can make it very obvious they like a particular girl as soon as she walks through the door. Sometimes the provocative dress sense of some girls can catch the whole gym unaware. I've found myself turning, glaring and thinking wow, I really can see everything, including what she's had for breakfast! It doesn't always go whereby the busier the PT the better they are. They may simply be a great salesperson with the gift of the gab. The key importance for me is the attention that the paying clients should be receiving from these 'dodgy' PTs, even if all they get is a so-called professional who simply does a countdown from ten to one in a droning manner while executing each move. It can sometimes sound a bit like listening to the numbers game in 'Countdown'. Let the client count for themselves, work on their technique!

If it's not lack of attention, it's lack of thought for the client. If you're in the gym for a considerable period of time, you might notice a PT who trains several clients back to back giving them the same routine. There's grandma, muscleman, skinny boy and Pilates princess all doing the same things. Surely somewhere along the line Pilates princess is going to get stressed over her bulky thighs, and grandma may give grandad a run for his money when he sees her ripped 'Madonna' arms.

I'll see trainers with their clients and look at them in this 'fitness-style glare'. Amazed at the exercise I'm observing, thinking I've never in my years in fitness seen that move; it must be a course I haven't yet been on. As I contemplate the move, I look at the victim doing the exercise and give a concerned smile to them. I try to remember their face, as I know I'll see them in my Pilates class the following day with backache of some kind. There's a need for 'dodgy' PTs to exhibit a 'you saw it from me first'-kind of exercise to other onlookers. The newest of new in trendsetting! Unusual moves used by PTs, which defy logic, are aesthetically intriguing to watch but anatomically crippling to perform. If you don't know any better, there's a general acceptance that this is how to get fit. Performing back bending moves like some Olympic gymnast gives the trainee a feeling of 'wow, I really am unfit, I must practice this more, and can I book in for another session with yourself as I don't know what I'd do without you!' When the phenomena of the Swiss ball evolved in the gym, PTs were clambering onto it like a kid to a new sweetshop. The classic squatting against a wall, and in some cases holding in a squat position, with the ball behind the back was something I thought, like time, had evolved but still I see it being executed in several gyms. Squatting to a 90-degree position with the legs takes a lot of strain to the knees! Not sure where it arrived from but probably some experimental magazine called 'Satanic fitness' and this gives more reason to the argument of why PTs need to constantly train and re-educate themselves perhaps through journals and not magazine hype.

Nothing quite beats the style of training one PT gave to his client. The treadmill was moving fast, the client was standing, straddled over either side of the treadmill with the trainer standing on the treadmill next to his client. Intrigued in watching the actions of the trainer as he demonstrated what he wanted his client to do, I thought I must angle my chair to get a better front row view. With the client's feet on either side of the runway, he was psyching himself by pacing forwards and backwards as if trying to time the speed of the belt, which was going at some considerable speed. All of a sudden he launched both feet on the moving tread with the intention of keeping up with the speed of the machine. Well, what happened next happened quicker than a whore to their client. He went down fast and hard! It went in slow motion – buckling at the knee as his hands tried to grasp the handrail at the front but narrowly missing. His hands braced for impact as they landed on the moving tread with what I presume would feel like rubbing hands on sand paper. His feet shot off the back of the treadmill in a rejected fashion similar to meat on a factory conveyor belt which had been given the red light. His bruised and battered body painfully followed his feet in the direction of the cross-trainer behind him, which someone was on. To add further humiliation and insult to injury, the gym was busy! The trainer looked stunned as if trying to work out where it all went wrong, or perhaps contemplating if his insurance documents were up to date. I didn't know whether to laugh or run over and help administer CPR. OK, he wasn't that bad apart from a dented ego but it was spectacular to watch and the devil sitting on my shoulder wished I'd filmed it and sent it in to 'You've Been Framed' for the chance to win £250. The poor guy, looking dazed and confused, was on his knees at the end of the treadmill as if praying for it all to end or perhaps thinking he should be on the treadmill now, not off it. He was apologising to the trainer as he thought it was perhaps a misunderstanding of what he had been told and thought he could have done better. I laughed to myself thinking of the sad prospect that some people really do put their trust in those they deem 'professional' without sometimes questioning the actions of their PT. A certificate of competence may be easy to achieve through oral, written and practical examination, but in the real world the volume of people with twenty-first century conditions a trainer comes in contact with means each session should be varied and focused on the individual and adapted accordingly, not the same thing for the masses. A simple tip for choosing the right PT should be to look at their credentials – where did they train, how long was their training and have they done further training since then to enhance their knowledge in a field which is constantly evolving. Also fire away at the questions to the PT for the reasoning behind doing certain styles of exercise. Educate yourself! Try a few different PTs within the gym to find which one connects with you on many levels! Trial a session first and never commit to a block of ten sessions unless sure the PT in question is the correct one for you and that they're not going to run away with your cash! The ultimate way is to chat to fellow members, as they tend to be brutally honest in regards to their own experiences! The changing rooms are the best for these types of conversational revelations.

A fairly busy female PT trained one of her older clients on a bosu ball (a half ball with a flat surface). She had him doing fairly complex moves on the bosu ball, which would've looked impressive even if it was performed by an athletic person never mind a sixty-plus-year old guy. The poor guy struggled posturally to stand on two feet never mind on an unstable surface. She eventually gave up on the exercise long after the guy did and did something a little more practical, like finish the session! The same PT in question came up to me asking what would be beneficial exercises for one of her clients whose back was steadily getting worse. Apart from wanting to buy her a T-shirt with the words 'KEEP CLEAR' as a warning to others, I briefly explained some basic pelvic mobility and stability exercises but advised that she would be better, along with her client, to take part in some Pilates classes to understand the concept. Even a basic movement can have a lot of technicality to it. I offered to spend five minutes with her client, not with the intention to poach him from her but to give him some basics. The PT met this with a whole lot of resistance. I'm presuming with the threat that my knowledge might actually educate him to get more from his back than what she'd been teaching. She wanted to meet over lunch and discuss exercises, but I declined. I wasn't going to design a programme for her to use on her client. As a freelancer, time is money, and besides, it's a great learning curve for her to actually think outside the box in how she could perhaps adapt her training style to accommodate those with injuries. If I did explain the exercises to her, she may have gone off and taught the same thing but achieved a different result as without proper training does she really know what she's looking for within a particular exercise? With this in mind, PTs can charge very different rates from each other. Should it be, the longer a PT has been in the business and the more qualified they are, the more money they should ask for? Courses can vary in duration. Some are one day long; others are months if not years long. One person may have ten one-day courses under their belt whereby another person may have studied one course which has taken them two to three years to do. Some have specialised knowledge, expertise and care to charge competitive rates. The new PTs in town tend to hear of the standard rate through discussions with their fellow colleagues and instantly match it regardless of whether it's their first day on the job! There are nineteen-year olds fresh out of PT academy copying their seniors, which I guess we're all guilty of doing but to charge the same rate as those more accustomed to the world of gym can be insulting to the long-standing PTs and the members alike. Unfortunately there is no standardisation within the clubs or the industry, so basically whoever qualifies as a PT can charge whatever they want regardless of level, skills, age and experience!

If it's not dealing with and understanding PTs on the gym floor or going into a group fitness class with the intention of improving fitness, health and wellbeing can result in confusion and feelings of needing to reach for the medical dictionary. 'Engage your core, suck in your belly and brace your abs' leaves the majority of participants wondering what the hell language the instructor is speaking. Nobody really questions the concept and will just follow the rest of the herd. This can be the same in a spin class where you may see many sweaty cyclists on a bike bobbing up and down doing press-ups! Why hasn't someone banned this ludicrous move whilst on a bike! It looks like an orgy of bike shaggers mixed with headbanging music to no real benefit to the upper body.

CELEBRITY TRAINERS...

With 'dodgy' PTs there closely follows the 'celebrity trainers'! I know a few of these so called trainers through having worked alongside them, and I guess some believe it's the next step up in the PT world. They've reached the top of the PT empire. It's questionable to when exactly the name 'celebrity trainer' is 'knighted'. Is it after coming in contact with a Z list (who are they?) 'Big Brother' reality-type celebrity, having possibly trained them once or twice? Is it once they have two or more TV personality / pop star people on their books that the name PT drops to become celebrity trainer? Changing a title doesn't give the individual in question any more knowledge than the standard PT. In some cases 'thick as shit' comes to mind with a touch of luck at being in the right place at the right time. Then again it depends if you want the hassle and demands of the celebrity in question. To me, hell no! It reminds me of my SRO days – a fancy title to a basic job of stacking shelves, except in this case the fancy title of celeb trainer is adopted to make the trainer feel somewhat more important in life. Living in London, it's common to bump into celebrities, and let's just say airbrushing does wonders! After seeing more than a handful of well-known faces it becomes a grievance of 'I hope they're not going to stop me from getting to where I need to be!'

Some well-known celebrity fitness trainers who have their own gyms in prestigious places within London have hired other PTs to work within their establishments. I come in contact with a lot of people on my rounds of many gyms and conventions and remember vividly speaking to a member of one of these so-called exquisite health clubs. They had terminated their membership after seriously damaging their shoulder and back through the training that was given to them. The unfortunate thing for the general public is that some celebrity trainers have opened up several gyms within London through the financial help of their fathers. For the lucky public, the pain and persistent misery is spread throughout! Appearances on TV, radio and other media channels can portray a confident celebrity trainer, which can cover up the lack of in-depth knowledge one holds. Money may buy gyms but it can't turn the intellectually challenged into Einstein!

Rates charged by celebrity trainers can be anything from £150 per hour and much more. At the end of the day it's lifting weights and exercise and if there are those individuals who have money to throw away then by all means do it. Some deserve the money they charge. There are many highly skilled and busy PTs out in the industry who charge realistic 'REAL' prices for the purpose being served. If £150 is the price for a one-hour session accompanied by a postural and nutritional analysis, then maybe it becomes less of a piss-take!

I'VE DONE THE COURSE NOW THIS IS THE WAY!

I've come across many motivational, inspirational and open-minded fitness professionals! By open-minded, I mean the ability to look at concepts of fitness and nutrition from a viewpoint to change one's thinking! We go on courses to learn and believe what we hear and see! I've always believed that eating a variety of healthy food is the way forward but these days, what's healthy? Some chew on sticks of celery thinking about their next weigh in! Others eat McDonalds feeling happy for the fact they're eating a meal which has 'happy' in the title and for the fact they exercise thus having a balance in their lives! We're told to eat fruit and vegetables in abundance, however most produce is often affected by chemicals to help promote quicker growth so that it reaches the market place in a quicker time. I'm open to supplements, but I'm also aware of marketing strategies trying to create a need within society that we all need 'this and that' for maintenance of our bodies and improved well-being! Now in an ideal world, we all would eat organic food and grow our own fruit and veg, drink plenty of water and exercise daily! In the real world, however, many, many people will never want the word 'gym' mentioned in their vocabulary! I'm often met with more confusion than I am resistance from the beginning, as in 'who's Jim?' or 'why would I want to torture my body and be in pain for days afterwards?' The fitness enthusiasts like the 'pain for gain' scenario and often pride the fact their legs are fucked after a training session with the S&M response of 'it feels good though!' Not everyone is into S&M!

Affordability also creeps in to eating healthy! The lack of time in our daily lives force us to grab a coffee and croissant in the morning, a sandwich in the afternoon and fingers crossed we manage to muster up a nutritious meal in the evening! On a nutrition course, we may be educated to eat properly and in theory it sounds great! In reality, life gets in the way, even to the most regimented within us! Not all of us have time to measure out how much protein we are planning to eat for the day. In practicality, we need to consume supplements to give us that extra boost, that extra burst of energy! For those who are overweight and not interested in exercise, unfortunately the fitness industry doesn't even cater for them! If you're not prepared to exercise and eat healthily – forget it! It's an utter shame but this is the hard truth about the viewpoint of some professionals in the industry! How does the industry reach out to those who will never enter the fitness domain? We may preach to the masses to eat healthily and properly but what happens if that's impossible? It can be fruitless to try to change the behaviour of others, as it would be to try and tell an alcoholic to stop drinking! It'll only happen if the person doing the drinking admits they have a problem. Once this occurs, then the process of change begins! With fitness professionals, there is a dichotomy of those who believe in supplements and those who are completely opposed to it! The ideal world seeks non-supplementation through education, as balanced meals within the day should do the job surely! The realist observes individual differences and understands that education could be the way, but it's not always easy to educate everyone on the same level, after all people may hear a message but do they listen to it? Even when people know that they should exercise and eat a balanced meal but still don't, and that's many people who fall into that bracket, what is the solution to this kind of problem? The condescending PT will jump straight in with two left feet declaring 'eat a balanced meal, veg, blah blah

blah!' After all, the nutrition course they've just been on states this, regardless of the family of ten having a limited income!

DODGY MEMBERS!

For every 'dodgy' PT you find there are ten dodgy members. You know the ones who for some reason take a shower and like to leave a deposit. Now, I love receiving gifts, who doesn't, but when it comes in the form of shit, it's pretty shit. I've never quite worked out why shit in the shower. YES, shit in the shower! Welcome to the civilised world of the gym. Is it perhaps IBS, enjoying the shower too much resulting in the inability to pull oneself away from it, a case of OCD and the need to keep cleaning oneself regardless of other emergencies or some cultural way of doing things that I've never encountered? All I know is that I'm not, or never will be, picking up the pieces! Vile! Speaking of smells and wishing I had at times no sense of smell, the male toilets can be a horrific experience if some over-intoxicated blubber of protein mass has ventured in and literally dropped their bowels into the pan. There needs to be windows or some form of ventilation in the male toilets but with most of them stuck in basements it becomes a competition to see who can hold their breath the longest. The smells may increase global warming but with ventilation at least my nose won't burn as much when entering these restrictive areas of unbearable pleasure. Even deodorant doesn't quash the pungent aroma of brutality.

As soon as you enter the changing room, the imagery of dodgy people can be a challenging spectacle to the eye! An older guy in his sixties standing naked with one leg on a stool blow drying his 'bits' whilst bending over isn't my idea of a pretty welcome to the gym. Does a towel not do the job these days? Then there's the poser guy (believe me there are many) pouting at the mirror while breathing out heavily to tense his abdomen, which is covered in a fungus of hair. My recommendation is shave it to see it! Some guys seem to forget where they are, or I can only assume they feel liberated walking around stark-bollock naked. Drying off in a showmanship kind of way by holding either end of the towel in the hands and buffing their ass furiously as if polishing their shoes to military standard. Even worse if sitting down and they stand in front of you – dick water droplets flying into your face. My recommendation is dry off in the shower cubicle to save wetting the changing room floor and put pants on as quickly as possible so those in the surrounding area aren't offended by such small matters.

If it's not nudity that can pose a problem to some, it's dress sense. It can be a case of 'all the gear, no idea'! Is there really any point of wearing Gucci designed tops when sweating and working out? Some shorts can be a little too short especially when stretching on the floor and as for tight little numbers – well, let's just say for the larger than life person who wears spandex over their clothes, it just looks like butt floss!

I have always been intrigued at the people who check their abdomen out at the start of the workout and then check again at the end of the workout to see if their abdomen is still there. Results don't happen that quickly! The muscle may be a little pumped but it's soon going to deflate back to its normal size. This is a common religion for many a poser – check the abs! It's the same story for many a female at the start of their workout, who climb cautiously onto the scales sweating at the thought of an increase in weight. They look down with bated breath, nervously hoping the McDonalds meal they had the night previous will fail to register. I love to creep up behind them whilst on the scales, place my foot on the back of the machine and press down lightly to see their body's reaction of rejection to accept what they see. Funny for me but perhaps a subtle, brief heart attack for them. It's even better when I'm about to teach a class, and I can guarantee they'll lose the pounds in my class knowing full well they'll stand on the scales afterwards. Thankfully I've not met anyone gullible enough to believe that – yet!

With every gym there can be a weekly, or in some cases daily, dose of theft. Members and staff alike with light fingers will steal anything that isn't bolted down. Protein shakes from an unmanned fridge are favourites for the muscle-bound warriors. Shower-gel dispensers are decanted by those who bring in empty bottles and top their bottles up, even better if it's Molton Brown. Glasses provided at the complimentary juice bar can often go walkies with those who need to collect a set back home. The transfer of toilet roll holders to personal bags and removal of mats and dumb-bells from the weights rack are just a select few items which can regularly go from the gym.

Most gyms have saunas and steam rooms, some have spas and swimming pools. It's a place to relax and unwind or in some instances, a continuation of the gym workout. Shenanigans in the shower cubicles, girl and guy, guy and guy or girl and girl having an intimate rendezvous is a common feature throughout the day and into the evening. Not always executed in the shower, the heat in the sauna and spa can get things tipping boiling point and allow one to lose one's mind or control of bodily functions. Well, if it came to a choice of rude goings-on or experiencing a hairy gorilla clip his nails or shave his beard whilst in the steam room, I guess I'd choose the loving frisking of two people, hands down, or maybe hands up in this case! Apart from seeing a large lady in blue shoes entering the spa naked, when testing the spa for cleanliness, the things found in the spa would make you think twice before entering again. Pubic hair, nails, tampons, urine and other bodily fluids along with 'parcels' (a polite way of saying shit) are a common find. I stopped using the spa for life after training how to test spa water and often cringe when I see people dipping their head below water level to surface and spray water from their mouths like some kind of fountain. Eurgh, yum yum!

As we can all imagine, sometimes it's not always the gym and its equipment that's the problem. When some people sweat it really can empty buildings. In one gym, a guy after a hard sweaty training session put his top back in the locker only to reuse it again later in the week. He only believes in washing it at the end of the week after session three. The smell is like an untreated sewer full of rats and onions, but on the plus side I've managed to strengthen my gag reflex. Has the guy in question lost complete use of his sense of smell? At least his sweat is absorbed within his shirt and not laying around like others! What is it with people being unable to contain, or at least mop up, their sweat after themselves? There are the runners on the treadmill with projectile sweat forcing me on every stride I take to duck to avoid the droplets that career towards me, and then from time to time I have to breathe over my right shoulder if the guy with the overused, unwashed shirt runs on the left of me. I dread the day when I'm running full pelt with stinker and sprinkler either side of me. There should be an 'in case of emergency' button on the treadmill for oxygen masks to drop down to help breathing when oxygen is restricted, like airplanes. There's smelling like a dog after a curry, and then there are those who seem to think wearing perfume whilst exercising is the way forward. Wrong! People, we're not there to smell good! If you're a stinker, whether it's perfumed or body odour, then train when it's quiet to minimise gym trauma to others.

STYLES OF TRAINING...

There can be various styles of training to achieve the desired results if performed correctly with a sense of control and understanding. Control in regards to the pace of the movement and understanding as to why the hell am I doing this exercise! Unfortunately many people have no idea why they're doing a particular exercise never mind how to do it. Copying from a fellow exerciser or trainer, mimicking the latest fitness magazine they've read or in some cases designing a move that is anatomically impossible with what they deem is the correct way to exercise. Watching from afar can be entertaining and challenging to the spectators' eyes. It can be as simple as watching the person on a treadmill at a moderate incline holding on to the panel in front for dear life while they power walk. With every stride, you can see the jerking and ripping of the shoulders as they struggle to keep up with the pace. Worse still and I've never understood this but reading a magazine which is placed on the console panel while jogging. Is it a picture book, as they surely can't read the words? I remember it well, a woman jogging on the treadmill with a sweater on. As she got warmer, she decided to remove her top whilst jogging. She grabbed the base of her jumper and pulled it up and over her head and it was at this point it appeared to stick. So with two arms in the air and jumper over face, the woman was propelled off the treadmill. At first there's panic, hoping she's all right, then the stifled laughter starts throughout the gym. Take the walk of shame! Treadmill workouts themselves can be varied whether it is the 'pushed for time' exerciser who lifts weights whilst walking or the woman who at every two-minute or so intervals keeps raising her left arm! Is she training to flag down a taxi?

At peak hours, a row of guys with their mates tend to stand in front of the mirror while exhibiting the classic dumb-bell exercise in the free weights area – the arm curl. This tends to be a problem for them and everybody else watching them. We all know these 'bicep boys' love nothing more than training their arms. The unfortunate thing for them is that they neglect other parts of their body, in particular their legs. Looking at these grown men with pin legs can devastate the trained eye as they rock to and fro gaining enough momentum to lift the heavy weight they can't lift. Get these fuckers pinned to a pillar and get them to lift the same weight, and I swear they would probably have to drop to half the weight. I guess it's not aesthetically pleasing for the ego to lift the weight of a bag of sugar on either side though! What's amusing is when skinny guy copies verbally what muscle guy says to help the biceps work! Imagine large muscle guy 'pep talk' his bicep during each repetition with the encouraging cries of, 'Come on bicep, come on!' Same scenario but replaced with skinny boy, 'Come on, bicep, come on!' There's a kind of hope in the room that he too will see the results of his hard labour.

With a concrete focus on biceps, sadly the legs machine, known as the squat rack, is frequently abandoned, and if a brave soul ventures over to attack the dreaded squat, it often looks a bit like a trembling drunk trying to get home after one too many. Once again, too much weight is added to the bar, which can result in a squat that resembles a Japanese sumo wrestler bowing to his opponent or a subtle bend with the legs as if some pole is directly under their ass. Heaven forbid if they go any lower, it may attack their legs!

The sit-up for the belly is regimentally done within every exercise session, whether it's in a class context or a personal workout. Watching people in general perform a sit-up can be exhausting as they move their entire body like a fish out of water. The sit-up can look more like a cross between a neck crunch and a fight against an imaginary shark on the floor depending on the type of sit-up being performed. The agony sketched on these dramatic performers' faces highlights how much effort it takes to work the abdomen. It can be a funny thing watching, admiring and impersonating 'the exercise face.' Veins pulse in the temples of the forehead, teeth gnarled with a constipated expression, eyes reflect pain or pleasure or both depending on the individual. Why is it difficult to smile during exercise? I've managed my facial expressions like I've managed my fitness, through training. Practising to smile while performing exercise to a group is an art form in itself as it portrays the impression of 'effortless'. Keep coming to my class and you too will enjoy the feeling exercise brings – euphoria! Faced with twenty non-smiling faces can make you paranoid with what you're teaching! I've taught and covered many classes with the thought of 'oh my God, they absolutely hate this, they're bored, I'm shit!' It's only at the end of the session that some people will approach me to thank me for the class and ask where else I teach! Phew! Self-esteem regained, ego reinstated! The most insulting thing to say to an instructor after they've covered a class is, 'When does the original instructor return?' So was the class really that crap!

Short of replying 'hopefully soon as you guys need a lot of work.'

Those who try their hardest to exercise while on a bike often get caught up in the moment whilst reading an interesting article in a magazine or a programme on the TV. The bike begins to slow in what must be an interesting part in the magazine or TV screen. In some instances it can stop! Some clubs I've taught in for years I've seen the same people doing the same exercises with the same body shapes. How utterly soul destroying! The same time, incline and speed is keyed into the machine week in, week out with an exercise face of despondency on the recipient. Losing the will to live, the frustration etched on the regular, non-achieving exerciser as in how to banish the ever-expanding love handles around the midriff. They know these machines can help them trim up but why is it not happening? A new plan of action is required. Stay awake during cycling! An increase in speed! An increase in incline! Perhaps a new lock on the fridge!

There are those who intentionally keep themselves at a particular level. A select few individuals who are able to achieve an advanced class continue to do the beginners' classes for two main reasons. One reason being the unwillingness to push oneself through laziness and the second reason for the fact they can feel egocentrically fuelled with how much better they're at exercising compared to their counterparts. Having an instructor reward you with compliments as to how amazing you are at being a first-timer can result in a nationwide search for all the beginner classes available in order to seek praise from all corners of the country. I guess we're all creatures of habit seeking praise and acceptance.

The idea of weight loss by many produces various phenomena. The larger than life soul approaches the trained professional to tell them they need to lose weight before summer. Unfortunately for most of these cases they arrive in the gym around May hoping that sometime in June the weight's going to magically drop off. It makes one wonder whether the weight loser has accidentally walked into the gym instead of the liposuction clinic. There's the guy who runs on the treadmill with his hoodie pulled over his head like 'Kenny' from 'South Park' in the belief that if he sweats profusely he will shed the pounds. In this day and age, people still have this misconception that a diet will help them lose the pounds. It will, but most if not all diets are not sustainable and deprive the body of much needed nutrients. The weight soon piles back on then the weight gainers response becomes, 'Well, I'm supposed to be this big, pass me the doughnuts!'

It can be highly frustrating for the avid exerciser who is belittled by the attitude of others who dispel their slenderness by luck and genetics. There are those who commit strongly to working out for many reasons whether it's weight loss, muscular development or purely to seek the benefits they reap from it. When guiding somebody in how to lose weight, I'm often amazed at how little is known on the subject! Just knowing that cutting down on fatty food consumption and to get off the seat from time to time will help! To question if fruit and veg is good for you is met with the jaw dropped to the floor in a kind of 'where have you been for the last decade'-type attitude! 'Do you not read books or watch TV?' Is there a sense of laziness to owning your own body and expecting someone else to do the job for you! The quick fix and classic questioning of, 'is there some pill I can take to slim down?' is heard time and time again. OK, there are the cases where weight is caused through medical conditions or injury but watching how some people exercise it's evident that laziness is the ultimate factor towards not progressing. A simple comparison of watching how a twenty-year-old exercises to that of an eighty-year-old can be very revealing.

Stretching, a neglected part of working out, is often the main cause for many injuries. A simple twist in a person who is stiff can throw their back out. Observing people's concept of stretching can be somewhat amusing. A quick push to the toes can be one's stretching programme covered before they commence their workout! I was doing a stretch routine in the gym one day when another guy noticed me and wanted to copy what I was doing. I advised him to go for simpler moves but it was like telling a dog not to shit for two days, it just wasn't going to happen. Intent on thrusting his leg high on a bar by climbing on to another machine to get his leg that high in the first place drew alarm to myself and other people around me. He then slowly lowered his other leg towards the floor so he was in a wide-leg stretch. I'm surprised he didn't rip literally in two as his upper body rounded awkwardly to compensate his inability to hold the position. It looked painful, but sometimes you just can't educate people in the principles of effective training. Sometimes it's best to let them follow their DIY manual. Lack of stretching affects most muscle-bound warriors who become tense and turgid with the inability to move fluently with each stride they take. This is, sometimes, seemingly the desired look. Embarrassingly there are the 'ego muscle makers' who regularly suffer from ILS (imaginary latissimus syndrome) or PCS (puffed chest syndrome). ILS and PCS, both the flaring of either the upper back or chest muscles and in some cases both, prove how much of a man one can be. The lack of muscle can be enhanced by a subtle postural change of widening the shoulders outwards to enlarge the back or squeezing the shoulders blades together to enlarge the chest. The only real cure for this syndrome is to actually work the back and chest properly by lifting the correct weight on the correct exercises.

Posers can be abundant in the gym when training. If it's not the sufferers of ILS and PCS, then it's those who stroll into the gym with the sunglasses on regardless of whether the sun's shining outside or not. These vampires venture over to a machine, peel their shades back just above their brow, pump out a few repetitions then either move to another machine, with sunglasses shielding their sensitivity to light, or leave. A quick pump is enough for macho man to then parade through the streets. It's either the shade wearers or mobile phone users that annoy fellow exercisers. Having to endure listening to a full conversation of what body part they're training, how successful they are in life, to how hot that bird was last night is from time to time rudely interrupted when the mobile phone they are using actually rings. I guess we are all eager to be centre stage from time to time but to what extent!

CHAPTER NINE

THE NEW MODERN GYM!

With fitness spiralling into a personal training culture, there can often be accusations flying across the gym when two people who are non-PT mortals train together. Gone are the days when the gym was full of fathers training sons, husbands training wives, mates training mates and other forms of training duets. In one club, a friend of mine was embarrassingly lectured by the general manager for training with his flatmate. As he coached and encouraged his mate, there was suspicion brewing amongst the PTs that he was some undercover 'outside' trainer. Bearing in mind, he wasn't wearing dark sunglasses, a hoodie with the hood up or scouting the room for security cameras! This has happened on many occasions in gyms, and I guess it's only fair too as the PTs pay a rent for the privilege of training clients within a particular gym. If it's the same two people training over and over, where's the harm! Unless they both suck at training each other, which let's face it is normally the case. Yes, there are those undercover PTs who sneak their own clients through the doors, but what can be done if they've both paid for access to the gym!

Some people are simply not interested in personal training for financial reasons. A large majority of people have eyes, and they can see the 'dodgy' PTs roaming the gym, chatting up members, full of guff and bravado! Some simply don't want to pay expensive rates to be observed on a treadmill, especially when there's CCTV in the premises. As for the mathematically challenged, they believe that they can count for themselves having attended nursery and don't need someone to do it for them. The vigilant members observe the PT's approach to the client, mimicking movements seen performed by those who know what they're doing and in some cases sniggering at the poor member for wasting their money on a PT who seems to not give a shit or have a clue with what they're doing. Everyone could benefit from a PT if they chose the right one. A few individuals do actually have a clue about how to train effectively without the need for a PT and in turn want to be left to train 'in the zone'. Some members, or in some cases a lot of members, are more conditioned than the PT. How does the oversized PT manage to clear a barbell past their belly? I guess avoid the exercise! How can an unfit PT possibly inspire an exerciser to run when they themselves gasp like an asthmatic whilst walking towards the treadmill?

With the PT rent steadily rising to around £1000 per month (in some places, more), there is increased pressure for PTs to convert members into clients. With pressure there follows strategies. Some use their physique, with muscles ripping through the fabric of the clothes they wear, to win over the muscle-starved wannabes and sex-seeking deviants. Some use their 'knowledge' by writing their memoirs on their profile boards demonstrating the courses they've studied, or perhaps in their head believe they're capable of studying. Some use their charms, wit and flirtatious side. Others read 'Men's Health' magazine the day before and replicate page by page every exercise to their clients! I teach in many central London clubs, and in one gym there was a member who had told me they had shifted over to another trainer because their original PT wasn't taking the sessions seriously. He was seemingly messing about in a 'bravado / knoblike' way with fellow PTs during their sessions. It was predominantly a gym full of male PTs thus a steady flow of excess testosterone. When these natural situations of swapping PTs happen, it's like watching two stags fight. Questions and accusations fly as to why one has poached another PT's client without due consideration to why the member moved over to someone else in the first place. If you're a great trainer, retaining clients should be fairly effortless! In some situations where clubs hold around twenty-five to thirty PTs there is the corruptive intent whereby the more confident PT will display to a member, who has a trainer, why they should actually switch over to them. Rather like mating season – flaring the feathers to impress! When the member is training by themselves the predatory PT will go in for the kill using their corrective and instructional skills to win the client around to their way of thinking. In some cases critiquing their fellow PT colleague's style and technique in order to put question and doubt into the trainee's mind. It's the underground world of the fitness industry where it becomes a fight for an 'everybody for themselves'-type attitude. As I've experienced the bitchy nature of fellow professionals, who seem to have the biblical answers to the correct ways of training, it's sad that information and knowledge can't be shared and explored with other like-minded trainers to enlighten ways of training for the greater good. They're not being asked to go on the Oprah channel and reveal all to the nation! Some just keep their cards close to their chest and refuse to reveal anything. It's like reading the magazines or statements made by the professionals to the 'secret' behind getting a six-pack or the 'ultimate' way to lose weight! Isn't it something we already know – get your hand out of the biscuit tin and into the fruit bowl! That being said, I've come across very enthusiastic and passionate individuals who share and push others in the same field to strive for a greater understanding. It's totally unprofessional to hear PTs slate other PTs within the same club regardless of whether they have a valid point to prove. Actions always speak louder than words.

Walk in to most gyms these days and you'll see many a PT hanging around waiting for their clients to turn up. In some cases the client doesn't show! Even though this can be intimidating for a first-time exerciser, walking in to what seems like the backstage of a gladiators' convention and listening to the conversations some PTs have can be highly amusing! Eat a strawberry, taste a strawberry; eat chocolate, taste the sweetness of it – what I fail to understand is when I see someone drinking a protein drink and then turn to their fellow counterpart to declare 'I can taste the protein!' Honestly! Next they'll be proclaiming to taste the atoms in the air they breathe! How on earth can you taste protein?

The average London rate for a personal training session is generally agreed to be around £50 for the hour. Some PTs, who struggle to meet rental commitments and household bills, stoop to a lower, underhanded charge of £25 in some places to get by! Perhaps it's how much they value their self-worth with the knowledge they possess! This unfortunately devalues the whole concept of personalised training by a professional, and then there is an expectation from the member for this rate to continue! Clubs set a suggested standard price for PTs to charge and for those who drop significantly below this is morally underhanded. Regardless if a PT is great or shit, sometimes a decision by a member to use one is made purely on what's affordable and what's not! It doesn't always go the cheaper the PT the worse they are, but when working in a club environment, there needs to be some kind of uniformity for fairness and equality to the rest of the team! Then again, similar to a supermarket having its value deals, maybe it's a consideration for gyms to utilise the shit PTs and offer value personal training at discounted rates!

Shouldn't the health and fitness manager from time to time be put through a training session by their clan of PTs to check for standards? However where do the standards of the health and fitness manager begin and end? Like many companies, PTs should undergo some undercover shopper to identify those who are wheeling and dealing, those who are sincerely legit to those who need to reread their personal training notes to clarify some key training points, i.e., turn up to sessions on time and use a diary for organisational purposes!

For many, fitness will never pay the bills! Some will leave the industry for full-time employment elsewhere, others will stick with it to pay off the expensive courses they've invested in and for a small handful they diversify within the freelance world and start doing fitness and glamour modelling or in some cases, stripping and porn. Those who survive the industry are those who are creative, perhaps not the avid watching DVD posse, but the DVD creators.

MOTIVATION...

As many members struggle to motivate themselves with going to the gym, some finally decide to abandon their membership after months pass and the realisation kicks in that they've not actually been. The discounted gym gear bought in January still has the price tag on it and will remain in the cupboard until it becomes a size too small and only useful for cleaning the floors, dusting furniture or dressing the dog! The regulars who attend persist with the same routine, which clearly has no effect on them physically and mentally by the looks of it. Faces of misery are caused by the monotony of repetitive movement with no results to show for it. Many large women in particular avoid lifting heavy weights with a fear that they'll become gladiators with a 'Shrek-like' resemblance. They fail to realise that the tiny weight they're lifting will have little effect on their bodies and will just result in more fat piling on and doors needing widening. It must be frustrating for those not actually seeing a change in their bodies as it's highly frustrating for myself and many other fitness professionals who actually care. A plan of action for the existing member or potential joiners of the gym could be to participate in two group fitness classes per week and perhaps a one-to-one personal training session from a reputable, affordable trainer. The majority of people need guidance in how to train effectively to attain the bodies they so desire or at least the ability to move more fluently with less pressure on bones and joints. Paying more for a personal training session doesn't always mean you'll get more! It's always best to do your homework and ask about or listen in the changing rooms for conversations people may have about their PTs. The changing room conversations, as I've said, can be the most insightful! After all, do you want your PT to talk to you or your breasts? Do you want to constantly be in positions that your gynaecologist wouldn't even ask for? Depending on your outlook on training there are those people who believe in the 'no pain, no gain' theory and others who believe in the 'train, don't strain' theory. Regardless of whether it's your first time or twenty-first time training, there can still be some form of discomfort the following days. It should be a feeling of having worked out with a slight ache in the muscles, not the inability to move for weeks on end resulting in having to miss weeks away from the gym or moving in a way that only spacemen move – one small step for man, one giant leap for mankind! If unsure with how the walk looks like, why not try shitting your pants and then you'll empathise with the inability to move freely!

Each visit to the gym can feel like repeating day one over and over in a 'Groundhog Day-fashion'; attend the gym, in pain for several weeks afterwards and thus avoid any form of exercise then hit the gym again! This is what sets apart the considerate, clued-up PTs from the downright clueless. I sometimes stretch and use the foam roller before teaching a class and whilst stretching observe my surroundings. I saw a petite female PT demonstrate an exercise on the cable machine to her male client. He looked like he had visited the gym a good few times and didn't look unfit. After her demonstration she then let her client have a practice. She kept the same weight she was lifting for him, and I thought fair play if it's just to correct his technique for the first few repetitions. However, the weight never changed and he continued with the same weight pumping out the exercise. It looked like a bodybuilder trying to lift a cushion! Hardly life changing! It was a simple case of what works for one person doesn't necessarily work for another. You have on one spectrum PTs punishing victims (ripping muscles as well as ligaments) and on the other side 'Mary Poppins' instructing a 'floaty' type session (open your eyes and now close them)!

Year in, year out the same patterns occur. By the end of January the gym becomes crowded with the 'New Year Resolutions' coming into play. The gym becomes a playground for the clueless. Clueless in how to exercise and in how to dress for the occasion. A clan of people who enter the studio for the first time have the thought of becoming fitter but rarely want to work for it. The lack of effort in each move makes me want to scream, 'Fucking work you lazy sons of bitches!' Some of the 'newbies' hold up the regular gym goers, as they require more attention through lack of exertion. Is it lack of understanding, lack of listening or just an overwhelming sense of lethargy, which makes the job in fitness demandingly tiring at this time of year? A plank / press-up position can look like a dog with both its back legs dislocated. This can be followed up by a whiny whimpering expression on the face of the overburdened individual as if to say this is humanly impossible. By the end of March, the bustle of the gym tails off with a small proportion attending on a regular basis throughout the week. The bulk of the population struggle to commit to three hours a week. Factors restrict us from making the time for the gym, but when we complain when our back starts to ache and a build up of lack of exercise starts to show on our weakened, stiffened bodies, we have nobody or nothing to blame apart from ourselves. I remember reading a great saying many years ago, invest in fitness now or invest in ill health later on. Lack of making time to exercise at least twice a week will soon force the exercise haters to take time off from work or worse time off from enjoying life. I know this only too well as I was a follower of the religion 'anti-exercise'. We make time for our doctor and hair appointments but for some reason find the ultimate excuses to avoid the gym appointment. I know all the excuses in the book as I creatively used them all up for avoiding physical education at school! Most of us don't care when it comes to fitness, but surely just being fit enough to anatomically move without creaking and cracking like some overused bed would be nicer. As long as we have the muscular strength to turn over in bed that counts as fitness surely! 'I rearrange the bookshelves, dance at the weekends and have sex frequently.' This and many other excuses I've heard as a justification to say I am being active compared to all these office workers who sit down all day. Active doesn't necessarily mean fit! After all, active smoking doesn't keep you fit (unless you're running with a fag in your hand)! I drink water regularly, which makes me visit the toilet frequently and the toilet's on the second floor. OK, excuse accepted as long as you're content with the effort you've given and happy with the overall result.

Gyms can be as exciting as tooth extraction but without the blood (well, in some cases)! Doing group fitness can be the cheaper option and allows you to blend into the crowd if you're not keen on the one-to-one option. If personal training doesn't appeal to you then make sure the class you go to is of quality not necessarily quantity. Try many styles of classes before you make up your mind which class is for you. For example, one style of Pilates can be completely different to another style and may be the difference to whether it's a one-off visit to the gym or you becoming a regular gym bunny! It may be a simple decision-making process over whether the instructor is inviting or a complete self-obsessed knob. Perhaps the 'eye candy' may be the reason for doing the class and if so, great. Get your ass into class!

If deciding against the whole gym idea and the choice comes down to books and DVDs then avoid those celebrity DVDs of overinflated marketing egos! You'll buy it in the January sales, look at it once then it just fills a space in the DVD cabinet for the rest of your life. Reading books can give you a start in fitness but will never be able to keep your motivation up. After a few sessions, strain occurs in the neck as a result of your legs being in the air and having to turn to look at the pictures in the book to see if you're doing it correctly. Before you know it the book becomes a handy place mat for resting drinks on! Boredom soon creeps in, and before you know it the process of thinking about joining the gym comes around as January nears yet again.

So if you're a member or planning to become one, unless you know what you're doing to achieve your goals, head for the classroom. Group fitness is the way forward and if you have a little extra cash to spare, invest in a one-to-one personal training session with a valued recommended trainer for a tailored unique programme for you.

REASONS FOR JOINING THE GYM!

There are many reasons for individuals attending a group fitness class: the oversized, cake lover who has come to realise that they are what they eat; the friends who team up together for moral support and to have fun; the housewife who feels isolated and bored at home and fancies a social life either through meeting new people in class or having an imaginary affair by seducing the beefy, bronzed combat instructor; the husband and wife team who help and support each other through the moves; the moaners who only love life if there's something to complain about; the first-timer, the old-timer, the fitness enthusiast all who are keen, or potentially keen, to work out; the performer / the exhibitionist who hogs the front space of the studio to either show off their new clothes, demonstrate how great they are or piss off the instructor for the fact they're always one beat or step ahead of what is being taught; the drama queen who feels compelled to groan with the simplest of movements or the thought of moving – oh, the effort; the comedian / the socialite who just loves to be around crowds and helps the class through the workout and often makes the instructor late (by chatting) especially when they need to rush off at the end of the session and teach a class elsewhere within the hour; the pregnant woman who craves to stay slim and trim in fear of the scales rocketing out of control; the injured who have been forced to come to class whether or not they want to otherwise suffer the consequences of the condition worsening; those who come to the gym to purely say they have been, but may not even exercise, or do as little as possible but still feel mentally satisfied as they have 'been to the gym after all' (I guess a coffee is a kind of warm-up!), and then there are the rest of those who attend the gym for a multitude of other reasons non-fitness related. Whatever the thoughts are on exercise and keeping fit, the only real conclusion is that it's a necessity for improving bodily functions like improved breathing and circulation. A large part of weight control is about what you eat! Eat a cake, be a cake! Combine fitness with healthy eating then the chances of lowering problems in the future are greatly increased. It's not rocket science! Well, to the majority of people it's not! If you like eating, then eat little and often! Exercise helps us burn the calories better and keeps gravity from taking its toll. So instead of having everything drag across the ground along with your feet, take time out to enjoy the benefits of fitness!

THANKS FOR COMING, THAT'S ALL FOLKS!

The last class of the week is done, the microphone is returned to the reception and the clothes are stripped off like some diver to their wetsuit. Hitting the showers after the last class of the week can be a rollercoaster of emotions. There's contemplation and reflection of the week just past, the class just experienced and the audience within each of the classes. It's a hard job working alongside others who are rude, emotional and contradictory. Instructors aren't mind readers, but to be successful, having some form of emotional intelligence will help to please around 75% of the class. Pleasing everybody is a mission impossible. Members come to class from different stages in their life, different preferences, goals, abilities and attitudes. As the warm water from the shower soothes the aching muscles from the weeks' worth of trauma, flashbacks of some of the performances come into mind. Did she really want to kill me with those dagger looks or was that her exercise face? Some do suffer from the natural occurrence of bitch face! In some cases, people are out for blood, not necessarily mine, but because I happen to be there all bubbly and smiley, I guess that could piss off even the happiest of people. 'Come on people, turn that frown upside down' or some shit like that! Navigating the ocean of opinionated students is tricky even when the customer is wrong, the customer is right. Will some people never be able to do a full press-up? Should I give up asking or trying and just tell them to watch and imagine doing it? Twenty minutes pass and I'm still in the shower concerning myself with options. Did I give enough modifications per exercise? I could spend a whole class modifying one exercise, and still the odd person doesn't get it. Short of modifying their face, the frustration whilst looking at them pondering is it rigor mortis, or are you really unable to move? Fluttering eyelashes, looking for sympathy is not going to work. Blinking is a movement but it's hardly going to get you fit! In some cases lack of movement could be a conglomeration of many things. Normally laziness is an overriding factor to avoiding a particular exercise, maybe it's clothing that just functionally won't move in a particular way without doing some mini strip-show, or maybe it's the baked beans on toast quickly digested thirty minutes before the class that is starting to surface. When I eventually get around to applying soap to my raisin-like skin, I think about those who love the corrective touch of encouragement and guidance. Their eyes convey a sense of 'touch me, touch me, touch me.' The eyes don't lie especially when they say 'don't touch me, don't touch me, don't touch me.' The 'don't touch me' eyes have a stronger ferocity to them – 'place one finger on me and I'll stab you with my eyes or smash you over the face with a yoga block.' The dichotomy of 'shall I touch or not' is blended with the eyes of frustration. Badly needing to get laid to the aneurysm about to occur with the rhythmless person next to someone can even confuse the most emotionally, intellectually-attuned instructors. What to do?

Stay at the front and don't move, hoping to connect with people through telepathy or walk around looking for those with puppy dog, pick me up eyes.

On leaving the gym, passing the studios and watching other group fitness professionals do their thing can bring a smile to my face and, in some cases, a tear to my eye. There's relief the week's finished and my mind and body can recover from teaching fitness. Stopping outside the studio looking in to the class taking place can conjure a reflective smile. Why do some instructors speak into the microphone as if auditioning for Broadway! Weird voices, like those on the rides at a funfair, reverberate throughout the studio. The part that brings a tear to my eye is catching an instructor at the start of a class shouting across the room over the microphone, 'Any injuries or medical conditions?' Is Helen, with pain etched over her face, really going to thrust her arm in the air and shout out 'Yeah, my haemorrhoids are throbbing like a bitch!' Well, maybe not quite as such but there are embarrassing injuries that people don't want to broadcast across the room for all to reflect. Looking at the faces of the participants in the class reminds me of my participants. Faces don't always tell the story. Attending classes to keep fit, to escape life, to perve, to socialise and the vast array of excuses we give to doing fitness give the instructor the daily challenge to approach the group on an individual level! Through love and hate, till death do we part! See you next week!

NOW WHAT!

So from uni, to SRO to fitness professional, now what? I've reached a point in life where I'm finally content! Well, as content as a human being can be! I found myself liking to be challenged in different ways and the world of fitness professional, which encompasses many roles, certainly does that! Whatever the perceptions of fitness professionals are, and they can stem from thick to highly skilled, be advised that only the creative and passionate succeed within an industry which is swamped with many creatures great and small, large and loud. Similar to the perception given to the professionals in the business we also have our perception of those entering our domain! The drama queens, the stressed, the disgruntled, the creatures of habit, the desperate housewife, the fashionista, the aspiring fitness professional wannabe, the introvert, the extrovert, the workers, non-workers, married, singletons, fit, not-fit, psychologically disturbed, mentally deranged to the physically challenged all help make fitness what it is! A creative challenge, but a life-altering fun one!